The Spirit of Healing

The Spirit of Healing

A Journal of Plants & Trees

by

Osahmin
Judith Meister

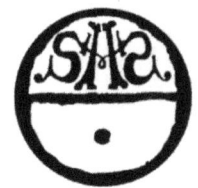

Ice Cube Books
North Liberty, Iowa

The Spirit of Healing: A Journal of Plants & Trees

Copyright © 2011 Judith Meister Osahmin

Isbn 9781888160543

Library of Congress Control Number: 2010940081

Ice Cube Books (est 1993)
205 N Front Street
North Liberty, Iowa 52317
www.icecubepress.com

Plant Photographs by Osahmin

All rights reserved. No part of this book may be reproduced by any means, electronic or mechanical, without written permission.

Disclaimer:
Ice Cube Books and the author offer this book as a source of educational information. It is sold with the understanding that neither the author nor the publisher are liable for misuse of the information provided. Author and publisher accept no liability for damage, or injury, caused by information contained in this book. The information presented is not intended to substitute for medical consultation.

Originally published 2004, Minaden Books

Dedication

"Migwetch," thank you,

to Keewaydinoquay,

"Woman Of The Northwest Wind,"

I place tobacco for your Spirit.

As you shared the way of Healing Plants

with the People of Today,

so I share the Teachings with

the People of Tomorrow.

May it all stay in Balance.

Acknowledgements

Many people influence a life, and a work of this kind. It is not possible to thank them all. I want to thank the Elders who were willing to share their wisdom about the Sacred Plants of the Great Lakes area, "Migwetch."

I wish to thank Jan Lawrenz, my friend and herbal associate, for helping me assemble this book. Her artistry and computer wizardry are responsible for the beauty of this manuscript. Thanks, Jan.

I also wish to thank my Editor, Carol Larson, for strength of character, for wisdom, and for endless readings and correction of my errant sentence structures.

Thank you, Carol, for your patience and encouragement.

Lastly I want to thank John and Donna McCreery for gifting the computer system to allow this manuscript to become a book. Thanks brother.

Table of Contents

FIELDS — 1

Plantain, 3

Chicory, 4

Lamb's Quarters, 5

Shepherd's Purse, 7

Ground Ivy, 8

Violets, 9

Strawberry, 11

Wood Sorrel, 12

Arnica & Calendula, 13

Corn, 15

Alfalfa & Ginkgo, 16

Pearly Everlasting, 18

Yarrow, 19

Mallow, 20

New England Aster, 23

Heal All, 24

Motherwort, 25

Catnip, 27

Nettles, 28

Mullein, 30

Black Cherry, 31

Dandelion, 33

Burdock, 34

Slippery Elm, 36

Curly Dock, 37

Milkweed, 38

Pleurisy Root, 40

Lungwort, 41

Sweet Clover, 42

Red-top Clover, 44

Hemp & Marijuana, 45

St. John's Wort, 47

Goldenrod & Elder Flower, 48

Purple Beebalm, 50

Wild Rose, 51

Sunflower, 53

Jerusalem Artichoke, 54

Sweet Fern, 55

Prickly Pear, 57

WOODS — 59

Jack Pine, 62

Red Cedar, 63

Hawthorn, 64

Sumac, 65

Black Locust, 67

Prickly Ash, 68

Aspen, 69

Hazelnut, 71

Maple, 72

Hickory, 74

Butternut, 75

Black Walnut, 77

Witch Hazel, 78

Raspberry, 79

Gooseberry & Grape, 81

Cleavers, 82

Cranesbill, 83

Wood Betony, 85

Partridgeberry & Wintergreen, 86

Spring Beauty, 88
Wild Onion, Leek, & Garlic, 89
Columbine, 91
Seneca Snakeroot, 92
Pipsissewa, 93
Stoneroot, 95
Canada Mayflower, 96
Bunchberry, 97
Solomon Seal, 98
False Solomon Seal, 100
Gentian, 101
Bloodroot, 102
Sarsaparilla & Ginseng, 104
Blue Cohosh, 105
Black Cohosh, 107
Trillium, 108
Trout Lily, 109
Wood Lily & Michigan Lily, 111
Bluebead Lily, 112
Indian Cucumber Root, 113
Evening Primrose, 115
Blue Vervain, 116
Licorice, 117
Wild Cucumber, 119
Cat Briar & Twisted Stalk, 120
Jack-in-the-Pulpit, 122
Golden Seal, 123
Wild Ginger, 124
Bittersweet, 126
Indian Pipe, 127
White Pine, 128
Red Pine, 130

White Spruce, 131
Hemlock, 132
Basswood, 134
White Ash, 135
White Oak, 137
Red Oak, 138
Beech, 140
Chestnut, 141
Ironwood, 142
Sycamore, 144

WETLANDS — 147

Willow, 149
Red Osier, 150
Balsam Poplar, 152
Crampbark, 153
Highbush Cranberry, 154
Tamarack, 156
Black Spruce, 157
Yew, 158
Balsam Fir, 160
Boneset, 161
Joe Pye Weed, 162
Marsh Skullcap, 164
Jewelweed, 165
Liverwort, 166
Swamp Milkweed, 168
Wild Yam, 169
Canada Anemone, 170
Horsetails, 171
Lady Slipper, 173
Calamus Root, 174

Bugleweed, 175

Skunk Cabbage, 177

Goldthread, 178

Bogbean, 179

Cranberry, 180

Snowberry, 182

Pitcher Plant, 183

Sundew, 184

Blueberry, 185

WATER & SHORELINE — 177

Water Arum & Arrow Arum, 191

White Water Lily, 192

Yellow Water Lily & Lotus, 194

Arrowroot, 195

Bur Reed & Bulrush, 197

Water Smartweed & Turtlehead, 198

Pickerelweed & Water Plantain, 200

Watercress, 201

Wild Rice, 202

Cattails, 204

Calamint, 205

Sweet Gale, 207

Silverweed, 208

Bearberry, 209

White Cedar, 211

Birch, 213

HOW TO DRY & STORE PLANTS — 202

FIELDS

We begin our walk at an open field. Some fields occur naturally, from the falling of trees or after a fire. Most fields now come from abandoned farms, leaving twenty or forty acres of land to be reclaimed by whichever plants are willing to take over after corn or hay crops. The wind carries seeds from plants who are well suited to filling the open spaces.

Where there is bare soil, Mullein explodes into the cycle. By the second year there are many neighbors; Violets, Goldenrod, Asters, Milk-weed, Grasses, and probably a few Rose bushes. These early settlers fill the place with seeds for future generations of themselves. Bare ground does not stay open for long.

If the area has rolling hills the plants choose the places on the slopes best suited for their kind of Being. Direct sunlight is the energy source for this abundance of plant life. As the tall plants fill in, they are joined by shorter plants who are then shaded from the full intensity of sunlight. It is not surprising that grazing animals come to the fields to find food. The birds may nest in the forest but the seeds of so many field plants are food for themselves and a nest of hungry children.

The plants must each devise ways to utilize sun energy without being burned or dried up from too much sun. Tall plants usually grow long, slender leaves to catch sun but not lose inner moisture. Some plants have thick waxy coatings on their leaf surfaces for protection. There are even plants who keep their leaves and flowers rolled up until the angle of the sunlight is less intense. I smile at the "ground huggers" who send their branches along the ground in the shade of other plants. They have tendrils, or sticky pods, to hold their stems on the ground. It is amazing how many Cleavers can grow sideways to fill a place.

The limiting factors of the open places are the amount of rainfall over the growing season and the richness of the soil. In a barren field it may take many generations of some plants to add to the richness of the soil. These "colonizer" plants then yield their space leaving the field to later plants who can outgrow them in the richer soil. It is not a total loss, as these early plants make many seeds that are carried by wind or by animals, to a new place to begin the cycle again.

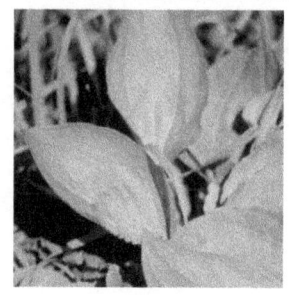

FIELDS
Plantago major

Plantain

Plantain is a very adaptable plant. It grows in the fields and just as easily in the grass of yards. It likes edges; the edge of a path, a garden, or a sidewalk. It has longish rounded leaves with parallel venation. It grows in a rosette without a stem. At the time of the seeds there is a long "rat-tail" scape covered with tiny seed capsules. In the language of the Native People of the Great Lakes it is called *"ceca guski buge sink"*—"leaves grow up and also lie flat on the ground." An Indian name usually describes the Plant, or mentions how this Plant might be of help to the People.

Plantain is a good first-aid plant. The fresh leaves make a fine antiseptic poultice for burns or cuts. What is a poultice? The fresh leaves are ground in a mortar (or chewed if you don't have a mortar and pestle along), then placed directly on the wound. Some people say "ick" about chewing a plant, but Plantain is worth the chew. Its medicinal gift is to neutralize insect venom! If you receive a bee sting or a spider bite, this plant really helps. The drawing action of the leaf poultice localizes the venom so it doesn't spread through the body. If the offending insect bites in the winter time, it is good to have some fresh Plantain leaves in the freezer. Dry plant leaves just don't work as well for a poultice.

Plantain is very cooperative for making salves. It has a high moisture content in the leaves and grinds easily into a green ooze. I have squeezed this green plant juice through cheesecloth and added the pulp free liquid to oil or cream for a burn salve. This good plant is analgesic (stops pain) and antiseptic (kills germs).

I am listing the Latin names of the plants so you will know exactly which plant to use. Common names for plants can be misleading.

There is also the challenge of hybrid plants, and I do not know the medicinal action of these plants. My herb mother was very serious about the way of medicine. She would say, "If you have not used a plant and think it might be of help to someone then you take it first!" This is why I feel more comfortable working with Native American Plant Medicines. These remedies were tested by people over thousands of years. I do caution you about sampling unidentified plants. Some plants may be very toxic.

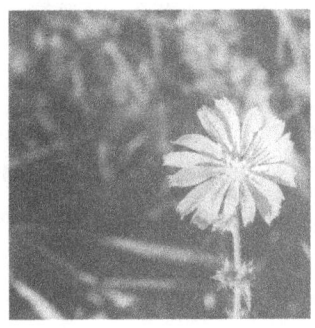

FIELDS
Cichorium intybus

Chicory

Chicory waits in the fields and at the edge of the road. Chicory grows to about three feet tall. It has an incredible root structure, and with time I think it could grow through concrete. It has basal leaves similar to Dandelion. What is most noticeable are the sky blue flowers with just a hint of reddish purple mixed in. There are many blossoms on each plant and this flowering continues through the warmest days of summer.

Chicory can self fertilize, or will accept the help of bees attracted to the flowers. The color and shape of the blossoms are part of the ongoing of the plants. An insect who helps with pollination is given rich pollen for its efforts. Plants are born knowing the wisdom of genetic variation.

Young Chicory leaves are good in salad, and if you can figure out how to get it out of the ground, the root is a good addition to ground coffee. I have tried this. Chicory makes the brew a little sweeter and richer. The root has so much good medicinal energy I save most of it for people who need its healing gifts.

There is a need to place an offering of Kinnikinnik (dry plant mixture) to say thank you to the plant for its sharing. Following the "rules for gathering" is an honorable way to collect plants, especially roots. I take only what is needed and make sure the plant can reseed the area.

A root decoction, which is one tablespoon of chopped root to a pint of water, is simmered for twenty minutes. This Chicory decoction is anti-inflammatory, antilithic, diuretic, and acts to lower blood sugar. It is helpful for someone who is borderline diabetic.

The most specific gift of Chicory root is the help for liver, spleen, and gall bladder problems. It helps the gall bladder produce more bile, helps release excess mucus from the stomach, and reduces uric acid which is the causative agent with gout, rheumatic pain, and gallstones. Remember that the best cure of all is not to get the "condition" in the first place. Find out what conditions might be trouble for you, and learn how to prevent them.

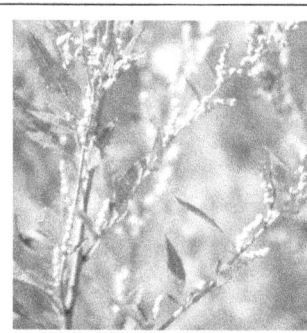

FIELDS
Chenopodium alba

Lamb's Quarters or Goosefoot

Goosefoot is a strange common name for a plant. It seems to refer to the shape of the leaves; wider at the base, coarsely toothed and narrow at the top. Anyone who gardens is familiar with this determined little annual plant that comes up from seed every year. A gardener may pull it out never realizing what a fine plant this is. The top of the leaf is green, the underside is whitish and fuzzy (perhaps like a lamb's wool). If it reaches maturity, Lamb's Quarters produces incredible amounts of tiny little seeds at the tops of its branches.

I gather leaves from the young plants for greens and prepare them like spinach leaves. My grandmother gathered the seeds in fall and cooked them as a kind of hot cereal with good protein. With just a whisper of maple syrup this is very good. Some of the seeds she dried and ground as a flour for breads. I tell you about this because this plant has a long history of providing food for people. Perhaps it is a part of our connection to the Earth…to eat the food that grows naturally where you live.

The leaves are high in iron, calcium, protein, and Vitamins A, B, and C. The Native People may not have named the vitamins, but they knew what kept them healthy and strong. The early colonists arrived in America with scurvy and rickets. It is fortunate for the colonists the Native People were willing to share food with them. I try to remember at Thanksgiving that the potatoes, wild rice, squash, corn, and beans were already under cultivation here (so was the turkey). If the *Mayflower* took them back to Europe they were probably listed as "alien" foodstuffs.

Please bear with me for a few moments talk about "societies." The Native People shared food with those who were in need. Their annual "Thanksgiving" ceremony was actually a meeting of the People to be sure all families had enough food to make it through the winter. If a family needed more it was provided by others in the village. It is only recent society which has found a way to "lock up the food." It is true, we depend on the grocery store, and they insist on receiving money…no money, no food!

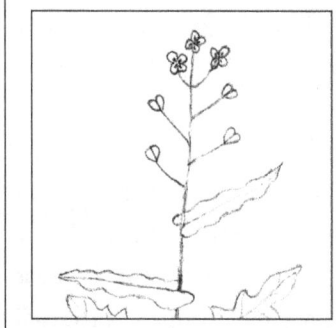

FIELDS
Capsella bursa-pastoris

Shepherd's Purse

As you walk through an old farm field, it is time to look for **Shepherd's Purse.** This is an annual growing up to twenty inches tall. If you have noticed this fascinating plant, it was probably the seed pods that got your attention. They are flattened, heart shaped capsules. Like the first two plants, this plant also has a rosette of basal leaves.

Shepherd's Purse is self-fertilized and doesn't ask help from any creatures to get the job done. The tiny white flowers grow from a slender stalk which later supports the seed pods. The size of the plant depends on the richness of the soil. Shepherd's Purse prefers the places where the ground has been disturbed.

This plant has many medicinal gifts. It is a good plant to dry for your family. Put down an offering of kinnik, or tobacco, or even a hair from your head, something to acknowledge the plant with a personal gift to says thanks. Yes, I really do this. It is a good way to ask the plant for its "gift of healing."

Shepherd's purse is anti-inflammatory and a gentle diuretic for water retention due to kidney problems. The tea, or infusion, is also astringent and can help with internal bleeding.

The fresh plant is styptic and makes a very good field dressing for cuts or scrapes. Sometimes wandering herbalists stumble into Raspberry bushes, or other plants which are capable of putting holes in people! This fresh plant poultice can also help with nosebleeds: just absorb some of the liquid with a soft cloth and apply to the nostril. If you are prone to nosebleeds, drink a cup of tea from the dry plant as well. Shepherd's Purse helps with the coagulation process. It is also vulnerary, which means it helps stop the pain of the injury.

Gather Shepherd's Purse after the seeds form and it will return year after year. The seeds are good roasted when added to a nut-bread or cookie mix, a clever way to put a bit of nutrition into an after school snack.

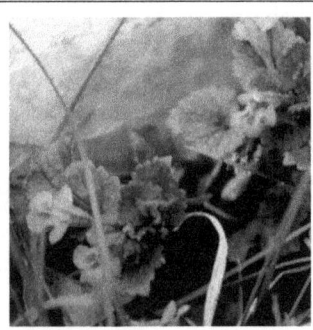

FIELDS
Glechoma hederacea

Ground Ivy

Ground Ivy is a vining mint with tiny purple flowers in the whorls of its leaves. It gets an award for having the most common names like: "creeping charlie," "gill over the ground," "alehoof," and others even less pleasant!

Many people curse this little vining mint, and are determined to yank it out of their yards. I wish they would send it to me! The hardest part about gathering this plant is finding a yard that has not been poisoned with fertilizer or insect spray.

This little mint is a medical marvel, what are we thinking when we pull it up and throw it away! It dries quickly, it works as a tea, and it even tastes pretty good. Ground Ivy is anti-catahrral (thick mucus), expectorant (productive cough), and vulnerary (relieves pain). To get more specific, it works to clear sinus infections and hearing loss from clogged ear passages.

What I use it for, at least most of the time, is for sciatic pain relief! This is a lower back or hip pain that bothers many of us who walk upright on two legs. To treat sciatica I make an oil tincture. I soak the fresh plant in oil for fourteen days. Any oil will do; like corn, olive, or grapeseed. I filter the liquid and use this as a massage oil wherever there is pain. It is an "in and out" kind of remedy; put the oil on your back, then drink a cup of dry leaf tea. When I do this twice a day, it really helps with the sciatica flareup. The same tea and massage oil combination is very helpful for arthritis in the hands. Many of our elders have problems with this condition. Ground Ivy is much less expensive than cortisone shots for pain and stiffness.

I like to gather this plant right after it blooms in spring, while the plants are deep green and lush. Some of the fresh plant I put in oil to soak, the rest I dry in brown paper bags. Gathering a lot of a small plants can be a bit tedious. Sometimes I try to trick my friends into helping me gather, a "bring-your-own-scissors" kind of party.

I remind you to use fresh plants for the oil, but use dry plant for the tea. Fresh plant has ten times the moisture content of dry leaves, you would need ten teaspoons of fresh leaves for a single cup of tea!

I always talk to the plants before gathering. These are "living medicines."

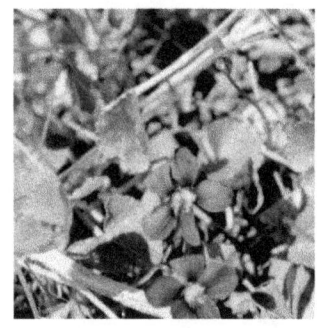

FIELDS
Viola odorata

Violets

Violet leaves are heart shaped with rough, scalloped edges. There are some very similar plants out there, so in the beginning gather the leaves when the plants are blooming. The flowers are beautiful little five petal blossoms that look like tiny orchids. If you gather leaves for salad it is good to only take one or two leaves per plant. That way the plant can easily recover and continue growing and flowering. Whenever possible, this is how I gather. It means moving around more but the plants appreciate it.

Violets come in many colors…blue, purple, pink, yellow, white, and sometimes combinations. They seem to play in exploring how many colors to be! The blue Violets are Wisconsin's state flower, a good choice.

I seldom discuss the chemistry of Plants, because for me it takes away the "actuality" of their existence. However, I will with Violets because they are being researched for a number of medicinal aspects. Violets contain saponins, flavonoids, alkaloids, and methyl salicylate. Those compounds mean the plant is anti-inflammatory, alterative, expectorant, diuretic, and anti-neoplastic. Oof, I know... anti-neoplastic means it slows the formation of new cells. Violets are being studied as an anti-cancer treatment. Methyl salicylate is an aspirin-like compound which is anti-inflammatory. Arthritis is a problem with the body's own immune system; it reacts to itself and attacks the joint tissue. Methyl salicylate can help the body with this problem.

Violets also contain saponins. Saponins are molecules attracted to water on one end and repelled by water on the other. The molecules travel along the digestive tract, spinning like little roto-rooters. Saponins in the Violets cleanse the intestinal tract, even the tiny pockets of the intestinal wall which can become infected (diverticulitis).

Our bodies are fascinating; they stay in communication with all their parts at all times. The Violets are expectorant which means a cough that removes mucus from the lungs. A cough can be treated by medicine that you put in your stomach. You knew that because that is where you put your cough syrup. However, as with all things we need to stay in balance, too many Violets will cause diarrhea.

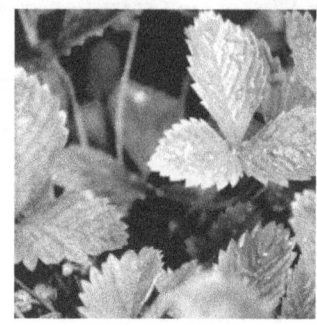

FIELDS
Fragaria virginiana

Strawberry

The wild **Strawberry** plant looks very much like the domestic variety except that it is smaller. There are three leaflets per leaf and they are serrated (jagged edges). The flower is white with five petals and blooms early in the summer. That is the time to gather leaves for drying. Again, if you only take a leaf here and there it does not interfere with the life cycle of the plant. Wild Strawberries are smaller than domestic ones, but they taste sweeter. It is as if the sugar is concentrated in the smaller berries.

Plants have many healing gifts which they will share with people, so it can get confusing for herbalists. The thing to remember is most plants have something that they do best. You won't need to drink a certain kind of tea for months to treat a condition. Violets are very effective to clear the intestine, Mints work well for gas, in the stomach, or in the intestine.

Strawberry leaf helps with bowel problems. It is safe for small children as well as adults. Funny, you wonder why we talk so much about intestines, they usually work well on their own. When they don't, you really want to know what to do about it! I call these teachings "what every mother should know," because it is never easy to know what to do for the little ones.

Strawberry leaves are a gentle tonic for digestion. Will it surprise you to learn they also help with gout and arthritis? There is a connection between improper digestion and certain kinds of arthritis. If the lining of the stomach or intestine is not healthy there could be a "leakage problem." The "clean-up" cells round up this material then have to put it somewhere. It appears that the open spaces around the joints are a tempting "dump site."

My herb mother always spoke about the "interconnectedness" of all things, and this is certainly true in the body. If one area has difficulty, it affects all other systems of the body. There are times when only a prescription medicine can do what is needed. Prescription medicines are powerful, but they are only a memory of the natural plant, or animal, that provided the medicine. A person may come home from the hospital and still be sick. A plant medicine can help heal the Spirit as well as the body.

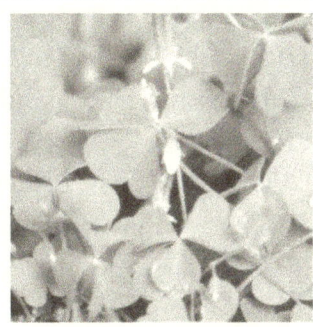

FIELDS
Oxalis acetosella

Wood Sorrel

Wood Sorrel is a fascinating little plant. It looks like a small patch of clover growing in an open area. I have found it near the place where the downspout empties onto the ground in my yard. Sorrel likes to share garden space, so I suppose it is easier for the roots.

Sorrel looks like clover until it blooms, when it breaks out in little yellow flowers not at all like clover flowers. There is another unique characteristic; the plant is sensitive to light changes. The leaves close up at night and just before bad weather. The Sorrel leaves grow on long, hairy stems. The leaves are divided into three leaflets as is clover. The Wood Sorrel is perennial and will come up every year if you allow it a place to grow. Sorrel grows in small patches, so it will not try to take over the whole garden.

The fresh leaves have a mild lemony flavor. Don't swallow the leaves as the plant contains oxalates that can trouble your stomach. Fortunately the medicinal sharing comes from a poultice of the fresh Sorrel leaves. A poultice of lightly chewed leaves is good for canker sores. It is not easy to heal mouth sores but this plant will help. For skin cancers I grind fresh Sorrel leaves with fresh red top Clover flowers. The healing action of Sorrel works well with the anti-cancer gifting of the Clover flowers. For less serious skin problems make a tea of the Sorrel leaves and apply this filtered liquid to whatever area of skin is problematic.

My grandmother combined Sorrel plant with fresh ground White Cedar leaves, using glycerine for the grinding liquid. (Yes, you will have to get a mortar and pestle, but such tools look good in your kitchen). Take the plant liquid from Cedar and Sorrel: squeeze it through a cloth. Let the juice drip into a small jar of skin cream and the result is an antiseptic, a wonderfully fragrant skin cleanser. Put a label on your jar that says "Sorrel/Cedar Balm" and share some with a friend. It is a fine gift from the Plants and from you.

When you make a medicine like this, the Physical and Spiritual healing energy of the Plants is included. Your good thoughts and human energy are a gift from your Spirit. Together these energies help with the healing.

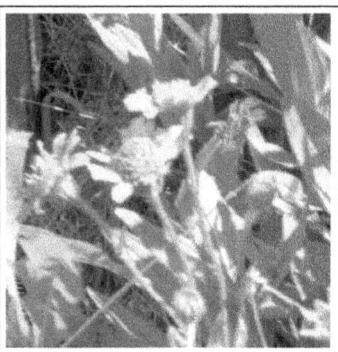

FIELDS
Arnica cordifolia

Heartleaf Arnica

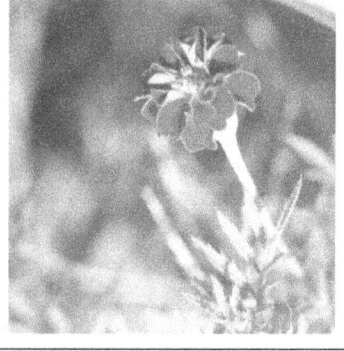

FIELDS
Calendula officinalis

Marigold

Arnica is a daisy-like flowering plant growing in patches along the roadside, or in fields where there is an opening. Each yellow flower has its own stalk. There are ten to fifteen petals per blossom, and each petal is notched on the outer tip. The lower leaves grow on long stalks out from the main stem of the plant. The leaves are oval with widely serrated edges and the underside of the leaf is hairy. As the leaf pairs move up the stem they get smaller and the top leaves have no stalk at all. This gives Arnica a pyramidal shape which is just right for catching sunlight. The energy for all the life processes of a plant comes from the light of the sun.

Arnica is not an internal medicine plant. Its healing gift is only for use on the outside of our bodies where it can be absorbed through the skin by sprained or bruised tissue. I tincture the flowers in a warm oil then filter the oil and keep it for use on strains, sprains, or bruises. You need to remember not to use this on open cuts, as the action of the plant interferes with the clotting of blood.

Remember to ask the right questions before doing medicines for friends or family. If the person is a "bleeder" this plant is not a good choice to help with bruised tissue. If Arnica seems a bad choice, but there is still a bruise or sprain to deal with, then use an oil tincture made from **Marigold** flowers. Yes, this is *Calendula officinalis*, the Marigold which grows in your garden. It is a lovely reddish gold flower and the plant itself turns away many insect pests. An oil tincture of Calendula flowers is also helpful for bruises or sprains, and it is also safe on open cuts. If the condition of the person allows, I will mix the oils of both Plants and ask for the healing gifts of both Arnica and Calendula.

FIELDS
Zea Mays

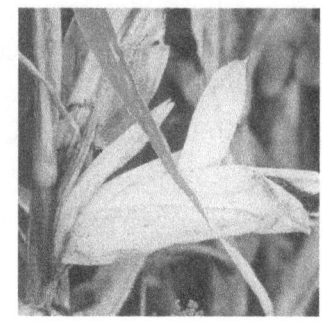

Corn

There are many, many kinds of **Corn**. Sometimes the kernels are almost white or yellow, black, blue, or red. One of the favored kinds of Corn which the Native People of Wisconsin grow is called "Calico," with many colors of kernels to justify the name. The People call Corn *Wickobi Siganug*, which means "turns sweet in cooking." How Corn came to grow here in Wisconsin we don't exactly know, but grow here it does.

Corn is a marvellous food crop, as it can be dried and stored easily for winter use. The People used birchbark makuks to preserve Corn for food and for seed to plant the next Spring. Some types of Corn are a kind of Hominy. The larger kernels are cut from the cob, soaked in lye water (made from campfire ashes), then washed and parboiled. If you have the chance to try traditional Corn soup, do so. It is wonderful. The soup is made from three kinds of beans and three kinds of Corn, with venison meat for protein. Corn soup gets better when cooking over low heat for hours.

The Corn plant itself is fascinating. The "pith" or center of the seed body is called the cob. Modified plant leaves form the sheath around the cob to protect the growing seeds. The seeds form in rows of thirty or more kernels. The filaments of the plant are silky and pale green when they first grow. After these fibers catch the pollen from the flowers, the silk dries into the brown threads we recognize on ripe corn. The gift of Corn is both food that is easy to digest, and the medicinal sharing of the Corn silk.

An infusion of ripe Corn silk is an herbal diuretic to help with gout or rheumatism. The tea is hypoglycemic (lowers blood sugar) and hypotensive (lowers blood pressure). Corn is an important medicine plant. Corn silk tea is helpful for uric acid buildup and infection in the bladder or kidneys. A gentle medicine is good, and it also helps with the pain and discomfort of these conditions. As with other medicinal teas let the Corn silk steep for ten minutes, then filter and drink. For medicinal use I suggest you buy organic Corn silk from an herb company. The Corn grown for food has probably been sprayed and that is not a welcome "addition" to your medicinal tea.

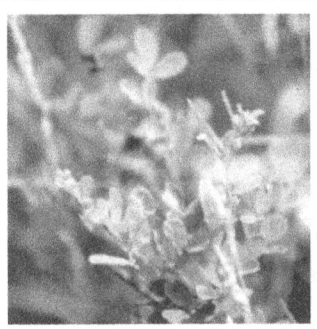

FIELDS
Medicago sativa

Alfalfa

FIELDS
Ginkgo biloba

Maidenhair Tree

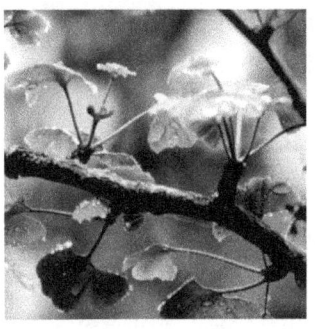

So, you think this time I have gone too far? This is hay! This is the neatly baled stuff we have fed to livestock for years. I do gather this Clover family plant. Although it is not easy to find **Alfalfa** that has not been sprayed, it is worth the search. It contains chlorophyll, carotene, and vitamin K. Somewhere in the spiritual mystery of this plant it also boosts the human's blood capacity for transporting oxygen.

Alfalfa dries easily. I like to gather it when it is blooming. Look for bluish-purple tubular blossoms, as this is when Alfalfa is at its richest. I crumble the dry leaves, flowers, and small stems, then run this mixture through a coffee mill (clean) to make a green powder.

This powder goes easily into gelatin capsules, two capsules a day is a good dosage. Alfalfa is helpful to the entire body in making more oxygen available to the cells. It is a marvel in that it also does this for the brain cells. Remember your elders.

Our oldest tree is the **Ginkgo**. Ginkgo leaves have been found in fossilized rock. It is still alive and well, and many cities plant Ginkgo as an ornamental along the streets. Ginkgo is pollution tolerant and will grow in almost any kind of soil. Ginkgo is the Japanese word for seed.

In late fall the leaves turn a yellow gold color, then one day (the tree decides when) all the leaves fall! I gather many bags of leaves, as a friend has a huge tree away from the road (pollution). When the leaves are dry I hand crumble them to store in canning jars.

Ginkgo has many medicinal gifts. It is a circulatory stimulant (helps with blood flow), it relaxes the walls of the blood vessels (the heart doesn't have to work as hard), and it improves blood flow to the brain (short term memory).

The best capsule ratio I have found is two parts Ginkgo powder to one part Alfalfa powder. Usually two capsules a day is enough. To keep the body supplied you have to take the capsules every day, the body does not store the Ginkgo. This is a fine plant especially for our elders. I encourage you to make your own capsules so that our elders, and those who need it most, can afford to take Ginkgo and Alfalfa. If your elders have stiff fingers, make the capsules for them, it is a good gift.

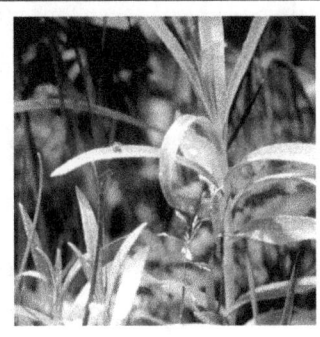

FIELDS
Anaphalis margaritacea

Pearly Everlasting

Pearly Everlasting is a plant about two feet tall that has pale gray-green leaves and stem. The leaves are long and slender as if the plant puts most of its energy into the blossoms. The flowers are clusters of small, white, round heads. The male flowers have yellow tufts in the middle of their white flowers. Pearly is a perennial, meaning it will come up every year and seed in more of its kind to form a patch or colony.

Pearly Everlasting dries easily and the little blossoms are very nice in Kinnikinnik. They help with ignition (caution, flammable) and burn well. The white flowers also look pretty mixed in with the other dry Kinnik plants.

The Native People used this plant for colds, bronchitis, and for headache relief. It was smoked or inhaled. We have become very concerned about smoking and sometimes overlook some of the medicinal or spiritual benefits. Inhaling recreational smoke is not a part of Native tradition. The Native People understood the lungs are the best contact with the entire body for certain medicines. The blood picks up plant medicine from the lungs and delivers it throughout the body. I am not suggesting that you "roll your own" just to get rid of a headache, but I will share what I experienced. A young man I know had a migraine headache which had continued for four days. He is a cigarette smoker so I gave him Pearly Everlasting leaves to roll. It only took four puffs to clear the migraine!

My grandmother suggested the plant worked well as a tincture. She said it seemed to help the body recover from stroke paralysis, but I have not tested this aspect. I have tinctured the leaves and stems and this has prevented cyclic migraine headaches. I encourage people to take the tincture before getting the headache. This is a better way if the headache is part of a monthly cycle. The migraine is a circulation problem in the brain; too little blood followed by too much. The headaches I have worked with are part of a hormonal or stress induced condition.

To make a **tincture** put dry plant in a canning jar, add equal parts of alcohol and water until the Plant is well covered. The Plant soaks for two weeks, I try to shake the tincture twice a day. About half a teaspoon per day is enough to begin the treatment.

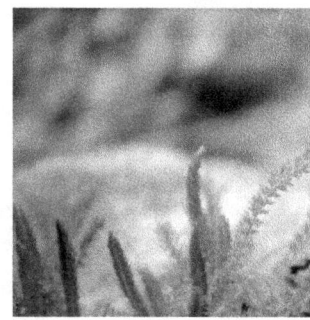

FIELDS
Achillea millefolium

Yarrow

Yarrow is a perennial, and it grows in clumps or colonies. The leaves are alternate, soft, fern-like, and very aromatic. Its flower is a white flat-topped cluster. Most distinctive of all is its odor. No other plant smells like Yarrow. For plants it is good to use all our senses, some plants may look alike, but they don't smell alike.

If I could only use one medicinal plant it would have to be Yarrow...it is magnificent! Yarrow is an antiseptic, both externally and internally. It is a good field bandage for cuts and burns. Internally it works for bladder infections or any problem in the urogenital area.

Yarrow also contains salicyclic acid which makes it a good tea for arthritis conditions. You can also tincture fresh Yarrow in oil and make a fine massage oil for swollen joints. Whenever the condition allows, it is good to use a remedy on the inside and the outside.

My herb mother made a Yarrow poultice moistened with glycerine to form a green, lumpy paste for young people with bad acne. It works to clear the skin even where it is pitted. The catch is the young person needs to sit still for twenty minutes each day while the poultice works. They also need to drink a cup of strong Yarrow tea to take care of the internal causes of acne. You can add a bit of honey to make it a more pleasant drink.

Yarrow is also diaphoretic, which means it will make you sweat. This is good for bringing down a fever, breaking up a cold, or lowering blood pressure. Anything that will remove excess water from the body will lower blood pressure, and that's what Yarrow does.

There is another fine gift from this plant, it has a slight numbing ability. If someone breaks a tooth at night, or on a weekend, you can pack the tooth with Yarrow to avoid the pain! This is a temporary solution for a tooth, but it does work. My grandmother told me that "fire walkers" would soak their feet in Yarrow tea before walking on the hot coals.

I'm not finished yet. Yarrow is one of the plants in Kinnikinnik. It is also used in a floral bundle to keep away negativity. In a Sweat Lodge there is often a bundle of Yarrow in the North for protection.

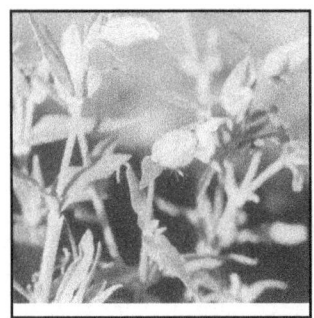

FIELDS
Malva neglecta

Mallow

I know, Spirit stuff. If it is possible to believe in "good" energy, why not, "not good" energy as well? And why not a plant for treating it? **Mallow** is at home along the roadside, in a field, or growing over a disturbed place. Mallow has an interesting nickname, it is one of the "cheeses." The name comes from the flat, rounded fruits that resemble a "cheese round." The plant grows one to three feet tall depending on the soil conditions where it grows. The plant grows upright with many branches. The leaves are rounded, heart shaped, with notches along the leaf edges. The leaves feel soft when you touch them. The notching of the leaves is continued on the petals of the flowers. Mallow selects a flower color from its palate of pink, purple, or white. These pretty flowers have five petals each and they grow out of the leaf axils (the place where the leaf stem joins the main stem of the plant).

This is a tasty, edible plant. I only gather a few leaves from each plant, so the life cycle of the plant is not disturbed. These young leaves are good raw or cooked. Mallow has a high level of mucilage, and the plant shares calcium and vitamin A. If the leaves are added to soup they are a natural thickener; no more "watery soup" for you.

The medicinal sharing of Mallow is in the mucilage of its cells. I do not know how mucilage benefits the plant, but it must protect it in some way. Often it is the protective mechanism of a plant which offers us a healing gift. A Mallow tea helps with coughs, bronchitis and pain in the stomach. These conditions welcome the coating action of mucilage. The coating is more than just soothing and protective, it also helps heal the lining of the stomach or lungs. This plant is also anti-inflammatory.

Let me digress a moment on inflammation. The immune system, which naturally protects your body, will sometimes get over stimulated, especially where there are allergies. The result is inflammation, the reaction of the body to its own injured or susceptible parts. ("Hey, that's not a germ, that's part of my knee joint your attacking!")

When the body is in balance the immune system works well defending against micro-organisms. This is a natural defense against harmful bacteria and a resistance to attack by a virus. You have probably been told by a doctor that there is no prescription drug that will destroy a virus, so you have it until the body is able to recognize and destroy the "invader." If you interfere with the natural immune system of the body, then you are more susceptible to disease.

I am not telling you to avoid prescription medicine, as the body sometimes needs this kind of help. What I would warn against are over-the-counter medicines we gobble down so we don't show the sniffles. This means we can continue working and not allow the body to rest and destroy the invading bacteria. It is interesting that many over-the-counter medications mask symptoms so well the body quits trying to do away with the germs. Suddenly you can only breathe well if you take the decongestants, or use the nasal sprays, so must keep using them. It is not a service to people when medicines are also big business. Now back to the plant called Mallow.

Mallow tea is a good choice as a tonic for the lymph system. This ductless system transports the defense mechanisms of the body and carries off dead bacteria and other unwanted material for disposal. Mallow is helpful for upper respiratory problems, swollen glands, sore throat, and the arthritis symptoms that seem tied to the body's response to a cold. For more serious conditions, like tuberculosis, herbalists have used an alcohol/water tincture of Mallow root. Tuberculosis is difficult to work with. It reminds me of arthritis, as sometimes the condition will go into remission, but there is always the possibility it will reoccur. This kind of situation would welcome a gentle tonic. Mallow is that kind of plant.

There is another plant with mallow in its name and that is Marshmallow; *Althea officinalis*. When the word officinalis is in the Latin name it means that the plant was once considered medicinal by physicians. It is the root of this plant which has the medicinal gift. Like the Mallow this plant is high in mucilage. A root decoction is helpful for sore stomach or inflammation of the digestive tract. (Yes, you have intestines, and sometimes they have problems). Marshmallow is a rather tasty medicine and is worth keeping on your shelf. Like the common cold, a flu-triggered upset stomach comes regularly to most people.

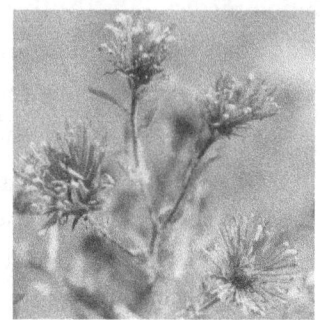

FIELDS
Aster novae-angliae

New England Aster

It is fitting that the common name and the Latin name of this plant are the same. **Aster** means star in Latin and in Greek. The abundance of purple flower heads with up to a hundred rays per flower are a wonder to behold in the late days of summer. You know the time; the grasses are turning a golden yellow color, and even the green grasses are a lighter shade. It is as if all the plants agree to put on this last glorious fling of color.

I do not use Asters for any medicine and yet I have affection for them. The caterpillars and butterflies find them delicious! The more sunlight that is available the more blossoms these plants produce. The shades of purple-blue shift as the forest edge begins to shade the Aster patches.

The Asters have sturdy deep roots that hold the soil in place, which is helpful in sandy places. The lower leaves are lance shaped and do not have stems, instead the leaves "clasp" the stem. The leaves get smaller as they near the top of the plant. Asters are self pollinated. All the rays are female, and surround a central disk with both male and female parts. The plant is perennial and grows in large colonies, and is well adapted to the open sandy meadows of Wisconsin.

The Native American babies travelled in a cradle board which could be hung in the low branches of a nearby tree. The motion of the wind in the trees was a comfort to the baby, and the dancing of many, butterflies around the Asters gave the mother time to gather Raspberries at her leisure.

Other species of Asters have white petals, or blue and even shades of reddish pink. You will find the Asters growing in company with many of the other plants that also like sunlight. Nearby patches of Goldenrod put out their yellow-gold flowers, and the Roses add their deep pink. It is a pleasure just to be in a meadow of late summer flowers watching the butterflies and listening to the contented humming of bees.

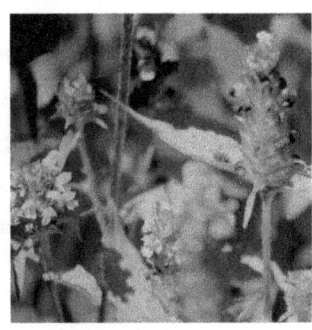

FIELDS
Prunella vulgaris

Heal All

I want to talk a little about Mints, the plants with the square stems, like Peppermint, Spearmint, and Lemon Balm. These are the ones we use for a pleasant sipping tea. The teas are highly volatile and need to be covered while they steep. They are a tonic and stimulative, good for circulation. The Native word for Mint is "oombahndahm" which translates as "to open up" as with *Monarda fistulosa* which is a breathing reminder for newborns. People used to say, "they get your blood moving." That is a fine gift, I only want to remind you not to drink them right before bed, because they are slightly a stimulant.

Just when you were getting used to recognizing "Mints" here comes a mint that doesn't have the square stem, but it does have distinctive features you can recognize.

The flowerlets, which are a purple-blue color grow out of a flower pod that looks like a green pine cone. After blooming the pods turn brown and look even more like misplaced cones! **Heal All** has opposite leaves that are oblong or lance-shaped. The plant doesn't have many leaves so I don't gather it until after it blooms. It is another plant to store in the freezer.

I know you are getting tired of poultices, but this one will draw out slivers! Sometimes glass or metal pieces are very difficult to extract, and Heal All draws them out. One of its Native American names means, "he draws out powerfully."

Heal All is a small plant with a lot of medicinal energy. It is an astringent (stops bleeding), antiseptic (kills germs), and is a local anti-inflammatory (keeps the swelling down). This plant is an excellent field bandage if you can't find Yarrow. Heal All also works well to dry up canker sores.

When you get more comfortable with the medicinal plants you can start working with some combinations. Heal All and Yarrow together, as a thirty minute tea, makes a fine gargle for sore throats. These two plants ease the pain, kill bacteria, and with a little honey, even taste pretty good. A child is more likely to try the sweetened medicine.

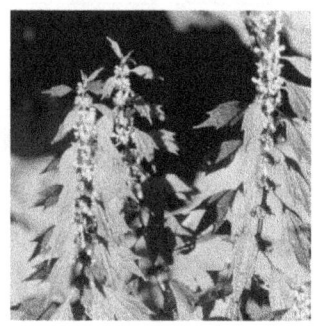

FIELDS
Leonurus cardiaca

Motherwort

Motherwort is an amazing mint. It can really get tall, up to about four feet! Just for fun it has two different kinds of leaves. The lower leaves are large, palmately cut into lobes (they look a bit like Maple leaves). The upper leaves are smaller, cut into a three pronged mitten shape with two thumbs. However it is the typical mint. The blossoms emerge from bracts along the stem where the leaves are attached. Late in the season the bracts dry and make gathering a difficult process (they bite!).

Whatever the dangers it is worth gathering the leaves of this mint. True, it is the strongest, nastiest tasting mint I have encountered. I dry the leaves to powder for capsules, or to tincture out in water and alcohol. I don't know of anyone who drinks Motherwort tea because it tastes good!

Before we talk about medicinal qualities I must state loudly, do NOT use this plant during pregnancy! It contains glycosides and alkaloids, and these are potent chemicals. The Latin name contains the word "cardiaca" which refers to its early use as a heart tonic. Yes, it acts to strengthen the heart muscle. It is also an anti-spasmodic so it will help prevent heart palpitations. Motherwort works well in combination with Hawthorn Berries. I have powdered both and put them into gelatin capsules for people whose family history indicates a weak heart.

This plant is also a friend to mothers. It is not for the child bearing years, but for the time of change when the symptoms of menopause begin. The Native Americans refer to this as the time when the "power is held within," rather than lost on a monthly basis. It is the time of wisdom, the time of the grandmother. Motherwort makes a great tonic, an alcohol and water tincture seems to draw out the best medicinal action for the symptoms. This tonic appears to act as a blood balancer and a nervine. The body needs time to adjust to the changing hormone levels of this time of life.

I prefer to gather Motherwort leaves mid season. The plants are big enough to allow harvesting a few leaves per plant. The leaves dry easily in a brown paper bag, and they hand crumble for easy storage.

Herbalism is a challenging task, it requires some learning. Herbalists need to "do no harm." I wish I felt as confident about the long term effects of prescription medicines. I am not saying avoid prescriptions, just ask the doctor to find the best and the safest.

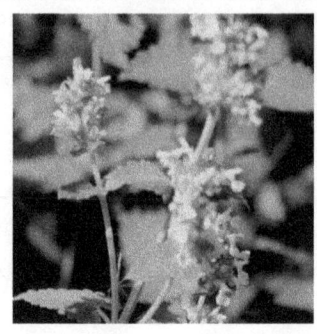

FIELDS
Nepeta cateria

Catnip

Cats do love this plant, it gives them a little kitty high. It is another mint, with square stem and jagged arrow shaped leaves. Each branch has its own flower cluster at the tip. You can find **Catnip** the same way the cats do, by its fragrance. It has medicinal gifts for people, so I keep it in my first aid supplies.

Like other mints Catnip is carminative (settles the stomach), but more important it contains nepetalone which is relaxant, anti-spasmodic, and most important, it will lower a fever. Young children can run a very high fever in a "minute and a half." Catnip gets right down to business lowering that fever. It is a nice tea that can be steeped gently for very young children, or stronger for older humans. It is wonderful, it works well, and there is no danger of Rye's Syndrome. Sometimes younger children cannot handle aspirin, as their body doesn't know what to do with it. Rye's Syndrome is very, very dangerous. Catnip tea in a baby bottle will work safely!

Catnip is a gentle, kindly plant. It helps with the aches and pains of a cold or flu, and it is slightly sedative. You can sleep and wake up feeling better! You haven't forgotten it is also anti-spasmodic. Coughs can be spasmodic, which is repetitive, and does no good for the body.

It is worthwhile to keep dry Catnip in one of those canning jars. It dries easily, and you need only gather leaves from a willing plant. The plant is perennial (you noticed) and will continue to share leaves for years. Catnip will grow almost anywhere. If you remove the grass that you now have to mow, there will be room for your medicinals. You don't have to pay for medicine that lives in your yard.

The Native American name for this plant, "Tsi Name Wuck," translates as "Big Sturgeon Plant." Strange name? I would like to share a different world view with you. The Great Lakes are markers for a land that was given to the "Anishinabeg" (which means "the People"). The Great Spirit guided them to this area and this is the "Homeland" for them. There is a Spirit of the Great Lakes which is represented by the Sturgeon, that huge prehistoric fish! The Native People felt such a Being could give important healing gifts to people (as well as safe travel on a large lake while paddling a small canoe). We forget that medicine in Europe was very primitive at the time of colonization. Many native plants are now part of American medicine.

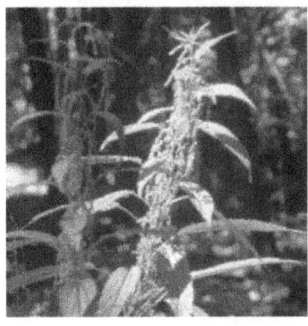

FIELDS
Urtica dioca

Nettles

A gathering bag or knapsack is a very handy tool for plant gathering. I keep an identification book, paper bags, Kinnik, and a knife in mine. The other thing to keep in the bag is a pair of leather gloves. Plants are very clever; they build ways to protect themselves from those who would eat, or gather them. Sometimes these protective devices are the very things which are medicinal in the view of an herbalist. If you touch or brush against stinging **Nettles** you will know immediately this plant is well defended. There are stinging hairs on the leaves and stem of this plant. The sting is a localized irritant, so if you wash your hands you can get the itch off.

Don't run away though, this plant is worth gathering. Nettles are a mineral supply depot. Nettles have human usable forms of Iron, Silica, Calcium, and Vitamins A, B, and C. The stinging capacity disappears when the plant dries or is cooked. The leaves dry easily and store well, but do keep them out of the sun as they lose color easily.

Nettle greens are very good in soups, the same way you might use spinach greens. As a tea it is a medical marvel; a year round tonic. It helps clear excess uric acid from the body, which is a blessing for those who have gout or other forms of arthritis. I use it also for people who get leg cramps from too much walking, running, or from humid summer days. Even the men will drink Nettle tea to avoid muscle cramps! Nettles also work well for internal bleeding, nosebleeds, uterine bleeding, even for hemorrhoids.

Nettle tea is also a blood builder. It stimulates white blood cells, aids coagulation (elders on heavy-duty blood thinners should talk with a doctor before using Nettle tea), and promotes red blood cell production. This is an excellent medicinal for people with anemia. Women have a tendency to a slight anemia every month.

The tea is rather good, as it has a natural sweetness. Those who need Nettles find them irresistible. It is good health for the entire family. Deer also love Nettles, and fortunately Nettles are vigorous growers and will provide for all the families.

Nettles are perennial, and they grow up to four feet tall! Some plants are all male, some are all female, and some are both. The plant knows which are which, I don't. The leaves are opposite, oval shaped with jagged edges, with a heart shaped base. The drooping flower clusters grow from the leaf axils. Nettles are a safe, healthy year-round tonic.

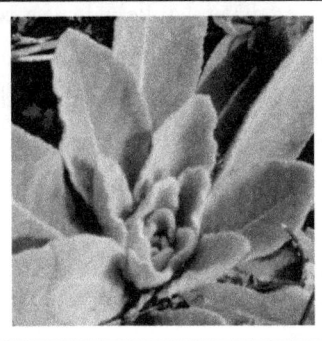

FIELDS
Verbascum thapsus

Mullein

Mullein is a very distinctive plant. Its Latin name sounds like you're trying to spit—*thapsus*. It's a biennial: its life cycle is two years long. The first year it is a wooly leaf rosette. The second year it sends up a tall spike with many leaves (still wooly) along the stem. The top is a long blossom area with many five petal yellow flowers.

This plant grows in waste places. It is one of the first plants to colonize a disturbed area. I tell you this as a warning. Plants draw minerals from the Earth. If there is pollution they also draw that from the soil. It is good for the Earth as a cleanser, but it makes doubtful medicine if you gather in a polluted place.

Mullein is an "indicator" plant; its growth pattern can be a warning to you. I have seen obvious genetic changes on some by the roadside or on trainside plants. A healthy Mullein has only one flower spike, it is not branched! I see Mullein now that looks like a branched Cactus, and I have to wonder what chemicals are there to change their growth pattern. What-ever it is, I wish we weren't putting it into the soil where the food grows for our children.

Mullein is excellent for bronchitis. It is an all-around tonic to the respiratory system. It is an expectorant (productive cough), and it is anti-catahhral (neat word that means thick mucus). Honey Mullein cough syrup is wonderful. You really can't overdose on it. It tastes good and it keeps the cold from dropping into the lungs if you take it while the symptoms are still in the nose and throat. It is very good for people with asthma, because it relaxes the swollen bronchial tubes.

I will give you the recipe. One cup of dried Mullein leaves to two quarts of water. Simmer, covered, for about half an hour. After cooking I filter the liquid through a clean, white cotton cloth. Cloth is better for this than cheesecloth as Mullein is a hairy plant, and the hairs should not be part of your cough syrup. The filtered liquid, which should still be warm, will dissolve honey. I put in about half a cup of honey, but you can sweeten it to suit yourself. The honey puts a protective coating on the lining of the throat.

The cough syrup will be both yellow and green. The syrup needs to stay in the refrigerator after this, unless you add alcohol to stop the fermenting of the plant proteins. Made fresh this cough syrup is good for children, but skip the alcohol.

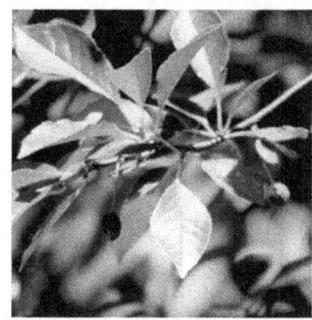

FIELDS
Prunus serotina

Black Cherry

This is a tree. Trees are plants, tall plants, and just like their smaller relatives they have a physical purpose and a spiritual purpose. My herb mother used to say, "If they didn't have a purpose they wouldn't be here...the same is true for you."

The physical purpose for trees is to hold the soil in place, to give off oxygen, to eat sunlight and use that energy to make life possible for other forms of life. Trees also make shade for other plants who cannot handle too much sun. The birds want me to mention that cherries are a wonderful food, but you know that. Sometimes the over ripe cherries ferment and the birds get intoxicated, (we aren't the only ones!). The seeds germinate after passing through the digestive system of the birds. It is a good arrangement for both species.

It is probably easiest to recognize these trees by their leaf forms. Once you locate a tree you can later see how the bark looks during the winter months. Cherry leaves alternate on the branches. They are narrow, tapered, and pointed with reddish hairs along the midrib underneath the base of the leaf. The bark on young branches is smooth, dark red, and very aromatic. Bring your nose along, it really does smell like cherries. Do NOT eat raw cherry bark, as it contains hydrocyanic acid (cyanide) which is neutralized when the bark dries or is cooked.

If it is poisonous why bother? With medicine there must be human caution, even a bottle of aspirin can be fatal. Many cough syrups are cherry flavored, this is not by accident. The spiritual purpose, the medicinal action of cherry bark, is to help the body balance the cough reflex. Yes, coughing is a reflex, you have no choice, you will cough!

Now let's talk about the bark of this good tree. Gather a few young branch tips. With a paring knife put a shallow cut down the branch (watch your fingers). Then cut around the twig at each end of the long cut. You can then peel the red outer bark off the twig. The pale green layer just under the red bark is the cambium layer. This is the part of the bark that carries the life liquids of the tree. With the paring knife strip off this bark, its rather like peeling a carrot. If you smell this cambium bark you will know that you have a cherry tree. Cook it or dry it, the inner bark carries the Spiritual gift of the Cherry tree. I put a tablespoon of Cherry bark in with the Mullein for cough syrup.

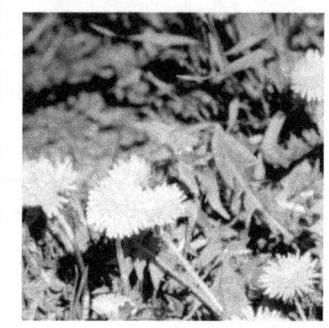

FIELDS
Taraxacum officinale

Dandelion

Dandelion is circumboreal, which means it grows all around the Earth at the same latitude. Not by coincidence it is used medicinally in very similar ways by different Peoples. I find this very reassuring.

The rough toothed leaves grow in a rosette and the yellow flower heads each grow on their own scapes. The plant itself doesn't have a stem. The flowers are edible. I have eaten them dipped in pancake batter and pan fried in oil or butter, yum. The young leaves are good as salad greens, but I don't always get out there to gather them in time. I dry the older leaves in a brown paper bag, then crumble them to use like parsley flakes on salads or potatoes.

What is medicinal about Dandelion? The leaves are a fine source of trace Copper. It is the mineral Copper our bodies need, and in a form that the body can assimilate. We need about as much as a few leaf crumbles will provide.

The root, yes, it is a lot of work to gather, but it is very good medicine. The root is high in Potassium and Calcium. A person taking medication for high blood pressure often loses Potassium which Dandelion root can help replace. The Calcium is good for bones. It is helpful for the elderly or those who cannot drink milk. Dandelion is a nudge to the liver and the gall bladder. It has been used to treat congestive jaundice and to help dissolve gallstones.

If my biological family had a tendency to develop gallstones, I would take Dandelion root to avoid getting the stones at all! Dandelion root is a diuretic, it helps draw excess water from the body. Okay, a diuretic will make you go to the bathroom more often, so don't take it before bed.

If you dig your own Dandelion root, wash it as soon as you gather it. A vegetable brush works fine. I spread the roots to dry inside a brown paper bag, and they should not touch each other. The roots shrink a lot as they dry. After about a week you can cut the roots into little pieces to use in a decoction.

A **decoction** is like making soup; simmer a tablespoon of root in two cups of water for twenty minutes. Leave the cover on the pan while cooking so that the water doesn't evaporate. Filter and store the liquid in the refrigerator, one tablespoon a day. Dandelion root is also part of an anti-cancer medicine which I will share later in the book.

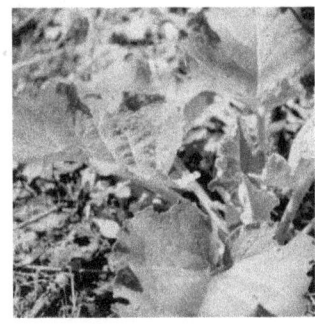

FIELDS
Arctium minus

Burdock

You know this plant; large lower leaves, and its flowers are burrs that stick to everything. These burrs are a good way for a plant to spread its seeds over an area, hitch hiking on other creatures!

Burdock is an alterative. Alterative means to change the condition of things. It is not a gentle change, and is meant to move a condition that is stuck. This plant is not a tonic, but I see people using it for everything. Please don't use Burdock as a daily remedy.

The part used medicinally is the root. Burdock grows big roots! I have found them two feet long and a couple inches wide. To gather you will need a shovel, or the wisdom to go out when spring makes it possible to pull them. You will probably get burrs in your hair doing this, so hopefully you have a friend who will remove them for you (primate grooming behavior).

Wash the root right away, then cut it lengthwise into half inch strips to dry. A thick root will not dry easily. When it is dry I chop the root into little pieces for storage.

Burdock is anti-microbial. It stimulates bile and digestive juices. It has been used for cystitis and to improve kidney function. It is a strong agent, cleaning the entire lower tract in a way that you don't need unless you are constipated. Most of all there is an internal cleansing that seems to occur on a cellular level. That is why Burdock is also used in the cancer treatment. Chemotherapy destroys cells in the body so fast that the ordinary cleansing systems of the body cannot keep up. The sudden buildup of internal toxins are a good reason to use an alterative plant like Burdock.

Another condition that might require Burdock is psoriasis; a dry, scaly skin condition. The Burdock root is prepared as a decoction. A cloth is dipped in the filtered liquid to place as a poultice over the affected area. The remaining liquid the person gets to drink (lucky them), about two tablespoons is enough. I would try this for seven days then see if the skin is clearing. If there is no change then try something else.

I worry about the people who feel their body is somehow "dirty" and want to cleanse it into submission. I wish I could say that sickness is only a physical condition. It's not. There is often a psychological entanglement which makes certain conditions very difficult to treat. If I heal a rash, what will a person determined to be sick replace it with.

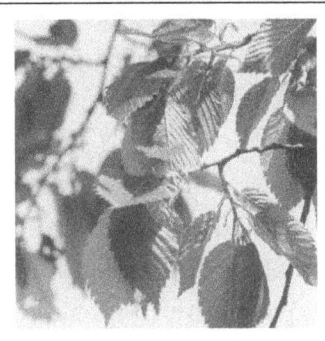

FIELDS
Ulmus fulva

Slippery Elm

Slippery Elm loves the lime rich soil of the Great Lakes. It usually only grows about fifty feet tall, but it is well adapted to the shady, wet forest places. The crown (top) of Slippery Elm is kind of thin and irregular. Okay, this is not the "best looking" tree in the woods, but like Jack Pine it fills an important niche. It mixes well with Ash, Basswood, Maple, and Oak, holding its own by producing both seeds and root clones where needed.

Slippery Elm blooms before the leaves come out. The flowers mature into disc like seeds which are wind dispersed. The seeds look like little flying saucers. The leaves are oval and sandpaper rough. These leaves are dark green, wrinkled, with red fuzz on the bottom side. The edges of the leaf are double toothed and the leaf bottom has uneven lobes.

The outer bark layer is rough with brown, corky layers. It is the inner bark that carries the medicinal gift. This inner bark is a slimy, fibrous layer that can be peeled in long strips. It smells a little like Licorice. Maybe that is why Porcupine is so fond of the bark. The bark strips can be dried and pounded (I do mean pounded, use a rock) into a flour-like texture for food or medicine.

The Slippery Elm bark powder is demulcent, which means it coats the lining of the stomach and intestines. This is a soothing gift for sore throat, ulcer and pre-ulcer conditions. Powdered Slippery Elm makes a nice tea, or if the person won't drink tea, it can be shaped into tablets for chewing. Either method will release the good medicine of this tree. You remember that Slippery Elm bark is one of four ingredients in the formula for cancer. Chemotherapy is very hard on the cells of the throat and digestive tract. Eating can be difficult and unappealing. Slippery Elm offers its medicine where it is needed most.

With a gift like this, I find Slippery Elm beautiful in its ragged, slightly scruffy form. This tree has found a way to coexist with our human, heavy handed methods of plant preferences. We do seem to believe that we, humans, have the right to decide which plants live or die. I'm glad the Slippery Elm over looks our foolish arrogance.

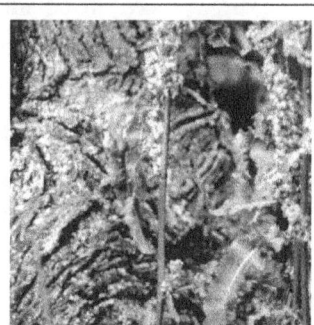

FIELDS
Rumex crispus

Curly Dock

Curly Dock is an annual; it starts over every year, which means it must be replanted, or reseeded every year. In fall I harvest some using a shovel. The Native People called this plant "Ozaawijiibik," which means "Yellow Root." The long tap root is indeed yellow-orange on the inside. When the root is removed I put in an offering of Kinnik and put some seeds in before replacing the soil. It is a good way to see to the ongoing of this plant.

Curly Dock has long leaves with wavy edges. Late in fall the plant turns a rich brown color. You may have seen it, as people use it for dry flower arrangements. The brown color is an indication of the high Iron content of the plant, especially in the root. The Iron in the root is in a form that can be assimilated by the body. Anyone who has taken Iron pills knows about this dilemma; you take the pills and what you get is constipated!

My herb mother used the root of Curly Dock for people with jaundice and those with anemia. To check for anemia look on the inner surface of the lower eyelid (be gentle). The skin color should be a healthy pink. If the skin is nearly colorless this could indicate anemia. Have the person get a blood test, especially if they are feeling short of energy.

Curly Dock is alterative, hepatic (kidney nudge), and a cholagogue (sees to balancing the blood). If the physical condition is mild then you do best to use a mild medicinal. Many plants overlap in their medicinal gifting. For mild anemia I use Nettles! I suppose I am protective of Curly Dock because it is another plant for the cancer treatment and I want it to be there for that condition.

The **cancer recipe** has a quarter cup each of Curly Dock root, Burdock root, Dandelion root, and Slippery Elm bark. Put the roots and bark into a gallon of cold water. Please, use a stainless steel, enamel, or glass kettle, anything but Aluminum! Simmer the plants in a tightly covered kettle for seven hours. Then turn off the heat and let it steep, covered, for another seven hours. Filter the liquid and store in the refrigerator. The dose is two ounces in the morning and two ounces in the evening. It sounds awful but it really has a slightly sweet, gentle flavor. I ask the person with cancer to prepare the medicine with me, because they need a healing relationship with the Spirit of the Plants.

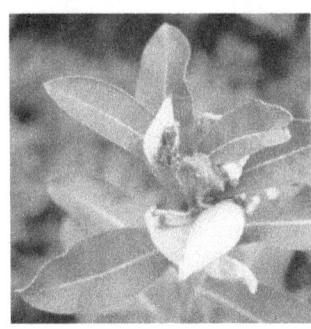

FIELDS
Asclepias syriaca

Milkweed

This is a perennial of the open fields and grows up to four feet tall. The leaves are opposite and covered with fine hairs. There is a sticky, white juice in the stem which probably accounts for the common name **Milkweed**. The purple-pink flower clusters are very sweet and fragrant. They can be eaten raw in a salad if you can coax them away from the bees who also find them delicious.

When the seed pods first form and are small, they can be boiled and eaten…HOWEVER…you will need to change the cooking water three times to leach out the glycosides! I prefer to leave the pods to ripen because there are cardiac glycosides in the Milkweed plant and I have great respect for the potency of such chemicals. As with other plants these glycosides are a deterrent to hungry insects, a form of protection for the plant.

Most often the plant was utilized by the People after the growing season. There are fibers in the main stem which were used for string, and this string was woven into fine mesh fish nets. Some of the colonists also used the fibers to make candle wicks. How does one get the fibers out of the stem? First put down Kinnik, then release the seeds from the pods (for next years Milkweed). Then remove the leaves and pound the stem gently with a flat rock. The outer stem cover will split and the threads can be teased out and spliced together into string pieces (it looks like monofilament fishing line). I have seen people roll the string fibers together and add to the length of string without missing a beat. My hands are better suited to making thin cedar ropes, but you may enjoy the process and have success with it.

Milkweed fluff is also good insulation material. It can be used for quilted blankets, mittens, even mattress stuffing if you find a lot of Milkweed. The only medicinal use for the plant is to neutralize warts. The fresh milky sap was applied to warts to stop their growth pattern. This is a sticky but effective treatment.

My affection for this plant continues into the winter months. The empty, or partially empty seed pods stay on the plant even after the snow falls. A clump of dry Milkweed pods makes a lovely fall display or photograph, if one is so inclined.

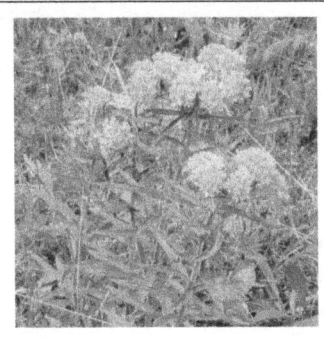

FIELDS
Asclepias tuberosa

Butterfly Weed or Pleurisy Root

Asclepias was the name of the Greek god of Medicine. It is fitting that this perennial, a genus cousin of the common Milkweed, should have that name. **Pleurisy Root** grows in the dry, gravelly, sandy soil which is common to the northern part of Wisconsin. The hairy stem grows to about two feet tall and the leaves are lance-shaped and alternate. The leaves are also hairy and colored a dark green on top and pale green underneath. Probably the most noticeable part of the plant is the brilliant orange blossom cluster. The blossoms usually host a number of butterflies who feed on the rich nectar of the flowers. In late summer after the flowers are gone, the long narrow pods form. The roots are a yellowish brown growth of tubers. The roots need to dry to lose some of the bitter taste, but this plant is good medicine.

I treat this plant with great respect, as it has healing gifts which are much needed. HOWEVER… as surely as you would only take one, or two aspirins…not a whole bottle, so you would not use Pleurisy Root as a beverage to drink for thirst on a hot day. In small amounts this plant helps correct the buildup of fluid around the outside of the lungs which is called pleurisy. It will also help with fluid in the lungs which is called pneumonia. Any plant which can help with these conditions is welcome. Pleurisy Root not only helps with the fluid buildup, it also helps relieve the pain of breathing that comes with pleurisy.

Pleurisy Root is diaphoretic, diuretic, expectorant, and anti-spasmodic. It is good to have a plant medicine that will help sweat out a cold or a more serious respiratory condition. I use Pleurisy Root as a decoction. For serious respiratory conditions I use both Pleurisy Root and Mullein. I prepare Mullein tea, with a quarter cup of Mullein leaves per quart of water. While this is simmering for thirty minutes I add a full teaspoon of ground Pleurisy root to cook with the Mullein. This decoction helps with the congestion and underlying problems of pleurisy. Pleurisy is a difficult condition, there is no easy medical solution for it. Anti-inflammatories are prescribed but Pleurisy Root can also help. The more intense the medical problem the more I speak to the Plant to ask for help with the illness—Physical help and Spiritual help.

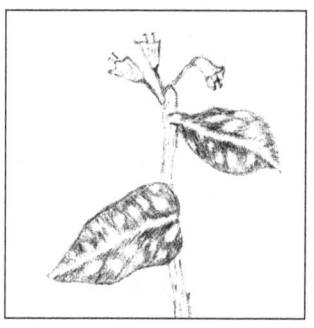

FIELDS
Pulmonaria officinalis

Lungwort

Lungwort is an unusual looking perennial. It grows to about twelve inches tall. The stem is bristly and the leaves have two styles; the lower leaves grow on their own stems, and the upper leaves are attached directly to the stem. The leaves are alternate and roughly oval in shape with areas or spots of transparency on the leaf surface. To me, the dry leaves look like some kind of seaweed. The flowers are funnel-shaped growing in clusters at the top of the plant. They are red, or blue, or both!

This is another plant called *officinalis* to record past medicinal use. The leaves contain mucilage, silicic acid, quercitin, kaemferol, saponins, allantoin, and Vitamin C. What does this mean? As you can guess from the common name this plant is specific in its healing gift, as its medicinal sharing is for the respiratory system. A leaf infusion is demulcent (soothing to lung tissue), and mucilaginous (restores moisture balance). This plant is helpful for colds, coughs, asthma, and bronchitis.

Lungwort also helps seal weakened tissue and reduces inflammation in the surrounding lung tissue. I have used this plant to help with chronic emphysema, though a difficult condition like this calls for the help of a number of plants. Sometimes I ask the plants for help and guidance in this kind of situation. If the condition had an easy solution the person would not be talking with me. Many times an herbalist is the last port of call when the illness does not respond to any medical treatment. Always in such matters, an herbalist must be careful to do no harm to someone already weakened. I check other resources to be certain the plants used are safe. Then the search begins, finding what is wrong with the person and which plants might be able to help them.

Certainly Mullein is helpful as a tonic to the respiratory system. As well, Cleavers to help the lymph system, Boneset for the lining of the lungs, maybe Ground Ivy for unproductive coughing, and others may suggest themselves for such a condition. An herbalist needs to know the ways of the body, the ways of the Plants, and in my view, be willing to ask Spirit for guidance and insight. What I am most certain about is the ongoing of a better relationship with Plants. They are willing to help if we ask in a good way and see to the future of their Children on this Planet.

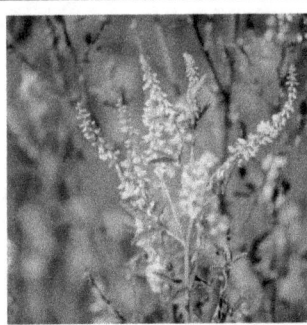

FIELDS
Chenopodium alba

Sweet Clover

Clover plants are tri-foliate, in that they have three leaflets per leaf. Sweet Clover is a tall, slender plant with dainty multiple blossoms at the tips of the stems. It is very fragrant, and the bees will tell you where to find this plant. It usually grows at the edges of farm fields or along the roadsides. The most difficult part of gathering is finding a place free of chemicals. I try to find abandoned farm fields, as they usually have Sweet Clover and many other wonderful medicinal plants.

Both yellow and white Sweet Clover are used as mild blood thinners. My herb mother put this plant into her spring tonic. Every spring the People of a village would come together after the long winter. In winter the families separated so there would be enough wood for winter fires and good hunting places for everyone.

In spring the women would joyfully gather newly grown plants, like Sweet Clover, who can share their leaves without injuring the growth pattern. The spring tonic would balance the blood after the slow-moving, sluggish time of winter.

Sweet Clover is a good friend to the elders. Their blood tends to thicken with age, no matter what season of the year. This means more work for the heart to try to send this heavy liquid throughout the body. Hence the circulation problems that bother many elders. Sweet Clover is a delicious tea that can help with this. I will give caution not to do this if your "elder" is already using prescription blood thinners.

When the plant is blooming I gather some of the long branches and tie them into bundles to dry (no brown bag!). Sweet Clover dries easily and smells heavenly. When the plants are dry I separate the blossoms into a glass jar to save for Kinnik, then crumble the leaves and small stems to be used for tea.

The mild blood thinning action of Sweet Clover is also helpful for menstrual cramps, especially those caused by overly thick blood in the uterus. I do hope you are not squeamish, some people are afraid of the inner workings of the body. The body is amazing, a mystery and a marvel. Like the Earth herself, the body has system after system to see to its balance and well-being. We who would be herbalists work to help the body with this balancing act.

Americans tend to over medicate. Artificial vitamins, minerals, digestives, nasal sprays, energy drinks…the list is endless. It is your own body that keeps you healthy.

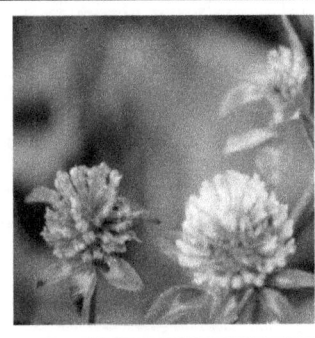

FIELDS
Trifolium praetense

Red Top Clover

Red Clover is a large leaf Clover with white markings on the upper leaf surfaces. It has large, pink blossoms at the top of stalks. The plant stem is green and slightly hairy. This is a soil renewing, "go with" plant growing in with Hay. You will find this plant also in the abandoned farm fields. The Spiritual (medicinal) sharing of plants is amazing. My herb mother taught that this Clover is part of the autumn tonic, to get the body ready for the winter months. It acts as a blood thickener and aids in the coagulation of the blood. That kind of statement drives the scientists crazy, they mutter about all Clovers being blood thinners. I only know what my herb mother said, and I have used it, on occasion, for nose bleeds. To do this I use a dry leaf tea.

What we do need to talk about are the blossoms! I take the infamous brown bags and a group of willing friends into a clean field to gather blossoms. This is the crawl-and-pick method. I am amazed I have any friends left. The dry flowers in a tea, or powdered and put in capsules, are an anti-cancer remedy. It is especially effective with cancer of the breast, ovaries, and the lymphatic system!

Let us consider this a moment. It seems Red Clover blossoms help the body fight cancer, which is very good. What I would suggest is those people whose elder family members have had this kind of cancer drink a cup of Red Clover tea each day to help the body avoid the cancer in the first place! Prevention is much easier on the body. The physicians say the genetic link for cancer is not proven, I don't know how you can prove it, I only know what I have seen. There is a tendency in families for certain problems to occur, problems like high blood pressure, early heart attacks, diabetes, arthritis, and (ahem) certain kinds of cancer.

The blossoms also contain salicylates (aspirin-like compounds) and flavonoids. I take some of the fresh blossoms to make a warm oil **infusion.** Take a double boiler (there still are such things), put water in the bottom pan, then put an oil (grapeseed will work) in the top pan. I tear apart about two cups of blossoms and add these to the oil (about one pint). I warm the pan until the oil is warm to the touch. Careful, you don't want to cook the blossoms! Let the blossoms soak in the oil for a day, then filter the oil. I have used this oil for people with arthritis swelling or for lymph node swelling. It works for both conditions.

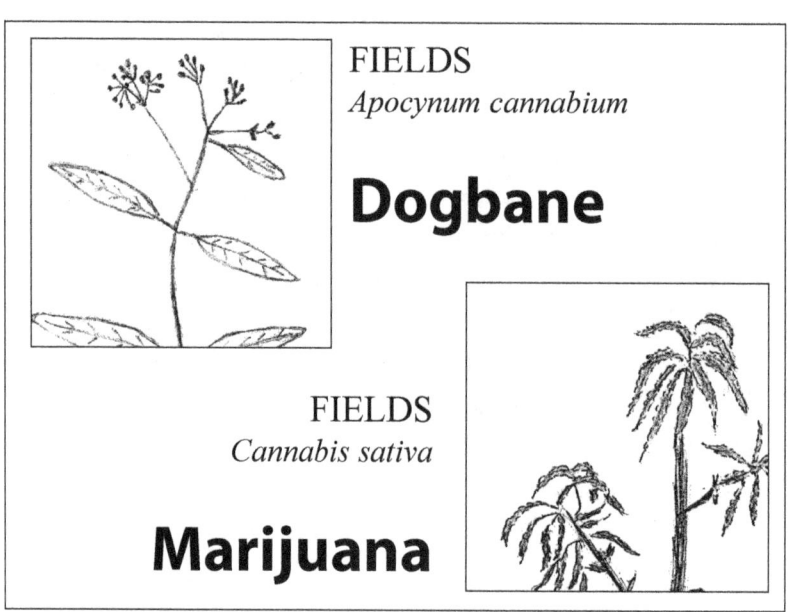

FIELDS
Apocynum cannabium

Dogbane

FIELDS
Cannabis sativa

Marijuana

I call this plant (**Dogbane**) by its genus name, *Apocynum*. This is a perennial found in open, sunny fields. Apocynum grows up to three feet tall and has a red, woody main stem. The fibers in this stem are native hemp and make fine cordage and weaving material. This plant has long, opposite leaves. The flowers are whitish-green and have five points. These flowers mature into pea pod shaped seeds.

Apocynum is related to Milkweed and can also serve as food and a nursery to the Monarch Butterfly. The Monarch utilizes the glycosides found in Milkweed to act as a defense against predators, as glycosides make their bodies poisonous to the "consumer." A bird only tries to eat this caterpillar once. You may know this story: there are non-poisonous butterflies who imitate the coloring of the Monarch Butterfly and thereby profit from the associated appearance. Apocynum is also toxic to humans, but there are other gifts this plant has to share.

A second plant of the same genus is *Apocynum androsaemifolium*, which is similar in appearance to *Apocynum cannabium*, but the leaves grow in whorls of four along the red stem. The blossoms are drooping, tubular pink blossoms which later form pea pod seeds. The milky sap of this plant was once used to treat external warts. We humans do not seem to be able to escape this phenomenon called warts, so it is good that there are plants to help with this condition. This plant is able to hybridize with another member of the hemp family...*Cannabis sativa*.

Cannabis sativa, whose common name is **Marijuana**, is a tall, annual native plant. It has palmate leaves with five to seven lobes. These leaflets are lance shaped and sharply toothed. Marijuana has small, green flowers that are male on one plant and female on another. I am sorry this plant has been labeled "illegal," as it is very, medicinal.

Compounds of Marijuana are used to treat glaucoma and the nausea which is an after effect of chemotherapy. In an infusion the plant is an antibiotic and anticonvulsant. It helps with pain relief, asthma, migraine headache and neuralgia. Far be it from me to utilize a plant medicine which offends the government! The upper plant and female blossoms have more THC. It would be better to use the lower parts of the male plant as a medicine, If one were using a "forbidden" plant as an infusion.

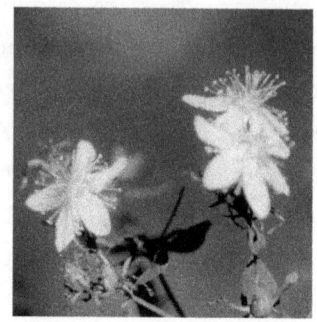

FIELDS
Hypericum perforatum

St. Johnswort

St. Johnswort likes to grow in groups, and I have seen entire fields of this plant. The plant has tiny opposite leaves that are attached directly to the stem, and there is no leaf stalk. The leaves have little dark spots on them. The flowers are yellow with five petals and many stamens clustered around a single pistil.

St. Johnswort has received a lot of attention from herbal manufacturers. They suggest it will do everything! It will do many good things, but not all it is claimed to do. I hope herbal companies will continue to plant and grow medicinal plants.

When I gather St. Johnswort for medicine, I wait until the plant has finished blooming, since the plant needs its energy to see to its children. I do not interfere with this. There is also an herbal guideline, "Don't take more than you need!" If we follow this then there will always be St. Johnswort growing in the fields.

St. Johnswort tea (steep for twenty minutes) is slightly sedative, anti-inflammatory, and analgesic (reduces pain). It works well for nerve pain like sciatica or neuralgia, which is pain in the side of the face. It works on the symptoms and the causes of these conditions. This same tea is also anti-viral, which means it can do battle with viruses. Very few plant medicines can do this. This is quite a spiritual gift, and why I hope most people will buy, gather, or grow their own St. Johnswort. I still want everyone to get rid of their lawns and grow their own medicine. It is pretty, economical, and you don't have to mow.

There has also been a lot of publicity about the anti-depressant activity of St. Johnswort. Yes, it does this, but it really only works well for mild depression which is likely to be short term. For more serious or chronic depression, it just won't be enough. St. Johnswort cannot be used in combination with other anti-depression medication because they work in different ways. Depression is very serious. I won't make the tonic for someone who is on prescription anti-depression medication.

Maybe I am being "over protective" of St. Johnswort, but I do want it to be growing in abundance to do battle with viruses which is its main spiritual gift. The last thing I want to mention is that all St. Johnswort medicines are RED! If the tea, tincture, or oil is not red, then it is not potent. It has not been prepared in the right way or with the right plant!

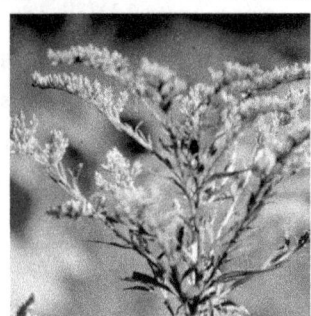

FIELDS
Solidago spp

Goldenrod

FIELDS
Sambucus nigra

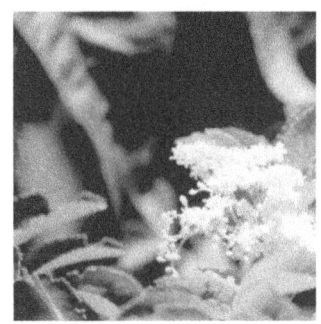

Elder Flowers

There are more than twenty species of **Goldenrod**. Be kind to them, because it is the Ragweed that makes you sneeze.

Goldenrod is tall with many lance shaped leaves. The most noticeable identification factor is the blossom; a yellow, triangular panicle. This is the part the Native Americans thought looked like a "squirrel's tail," and call the plant "Adjidamo Wano." The plants were named either by appearance, or by their medicinal action.

Some species of Goldenrod are very fragrant. There is a sweet smelling Goldenrod native to Illinois that I love to gather for Kinnik. Goldenrod does a fine job of reproducing with very little help from me. I do gather some leaves early in the growing season because by mid summer the leaves get a blight that is not good for medicine.

Goldenrod is a fine medicinal plant. It is specific to upper respiratory catahhr which causes a tight cough. I make a tea of Goldenrod leaves and dry **Elder Blossoms** which works as a cold preventive, as well as helping with a stubborn cough.

I would like to share a story with you, a story about a certain kind of butterfly, one that drives the scientists crazy! This butterfly eats Goldenrod leaves. Sometimes there are so many butterflies they eat up all the Goldenrod! When this happens a lot of butterflies die off, but some do not. They fly over and start eating Asters! Well, some butterflies say, "I won't eat asters! My mother ate Goldenrod, my grandmother ate Goldenrod, I'll be darned if I'll eat Asters!" Those are the ones that die off. The other ones who eat Asters then mutate. There is something in the Asters that causes genetic changes so that they can mate with a different species of butterfly, one that eats Milkweed! Their children can then eat Milkweed! This really does annoy the scientists, they don't think creatures should be able to change species like that. It happens, and plants are masters at creating new species.

We humans spend a lot of time trying to get the plants to do what we want. The genetics are altered to get bigger fruit, or an insect resistant plant. That's fine as long as the original plant continues to exist. Many seed companies create "hybrids," plants that don't reproduce. Then we must buy their seed…I worry about this tampering.

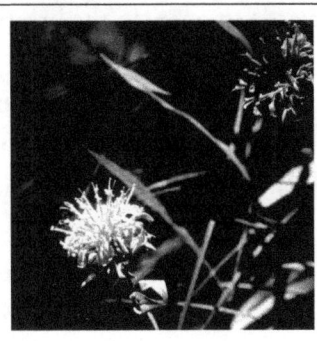

FIELDS
Monarda fistulosa

Purple Beebalm

At mid summer in the field we may see hundreds of pale purple blossoms. The bees are delighted and busily gather pollen for their honey making ventures. I usually call this plant Monarda and recognize it is a Mint. It has a square stem that is green early in the season, but turns a reddish brown in summer.

This is the "mintiest" of the Mints. Mints are vigorous colonizers and easily spread themselves across a field.

Like other fragrant mints, Monarda makes a carminative tea, it helps settle an upset stomach. It is also helpful for colic in very young babies. A tea or infusion, almost always steeps for at least ten minutes. I usually pour one cup of boiling water over the leaves, cover the cup, then filter after ten minutes. However, Monarda only steeps for one minute! I cover the cup tightly so that the medicinal aspect does not evaporate or escape because the essence of Monarda is volatile. My herb mother taught me to keep Mint teas in the refrigerator, because they work best medicinally when they are cool.

My herb mother also said, "some newborns forget to breathe, because they are new at being people and breathing is not a habit." She would cut pieces of fresh Monarda and put them in the top part of a double boiler, about one half cup of plant to one half cup of oil. She warmed the mix carefully above warm water until it was warm to the touch. She let the mixture soak, covered, for an entire day. After filtering there was a fragrant oil to put on the newborn's chest, a reminder to breathe! This oil is also an effective inhalant for adults who have congestion or breathing problems from asthma or bronchitis. It is the spiritual gift of Monarda to open up the breathing passages.

Monarda is also a welcome ingredient in Kinnikinnik. When I gather plants for Kinnik I talk to the plants to tell them what is needed. The plants seem pleased to be a part of the prayers and thanksgivings. They almost appear to be smug about the honor of it (sound of plants singing "we're going to be Kinnik"). Only the above ground parts of Monarda are used for Kinnik or for medicinals. This way the Mints continue being there in the field for butterflies, bees, and for me.

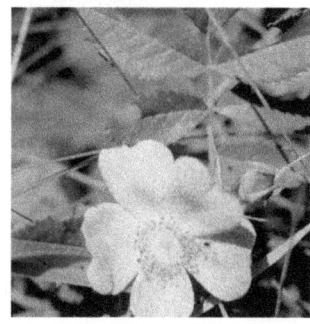

FIELDS
Rosa spp

Wild Rose

One day the **Roses** were gone! The animals were horrified, many of them needed Roses to survive. Quickly they called a Council to talk about this problem. Each species of animal denied doing anything to harm the Roses. *We are noble, we practice conservation. Don't we always leave fertilizer beside the bushes'?*

After many hours of talk it finally came out that the rabbits had taken the last bites of the Rose bushes. "We only nibbled the roots because that's all that was left, we didn't eat the whole bush," the rabbits tried to explain what had happened, but the other animals did not listen. "You admit you ate the last of the Roses, so we'll give you what you gave the Roses." All the animals pounced on the rabbits, yanking on their ears and pulling on their tails. The rabbits would probably have been destroyed, but a Manitou (a Spirit of that place) spoke up and told the animals to stop.

"You there, Animals, you all had a hand in what has happened. You, bees and butterflies, you took all the pollen from the flowers. You grasshoppers and caterpillars, you ate the leaves. You grazing ones, you ate the stems down to the ground. The rabbits only ate what was left. You must not destroy the rabbits!"

By this time the rabbits had very long ears, indeed, and only stubby tails. The Manitou continued to speak. "From this day on there will be protection for the Roses, they will have thorns to defend themselves against your greediness. This will mean some creatures will not be able to use the Roses, so some species will cease to exist on this Earth." The animals were ashamed of what they had done to the Roses.

This is an old story, I am sorry to say it is still happening today. We destroy species after species, and when this happens the Earth is less able to reach its full potential.

The Wild Rose is beautiful. It has a rich pink flower with five petals. It grows flowers first, then seed pods on its prickly arched stems. Every fall after the first killing frost, I collect Rose Hips. I hope you still have the leather gloves! Those little, fleshy, red hips are the best source of Vitamin C. They dry easily and make a wonderful tea. Rose hip tea helps prevent colds and other internal infection. Spread the Rose hips out on a paper bag and let them dry. Be careful to spread them apart. You don't want your good medicine to mold!

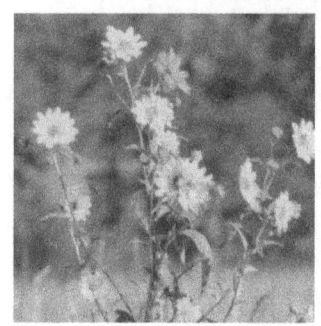

FIELDS
Helianthus occidentalis

Sunflower

Sunflowers may be annuals or perennials depending on the species. The word *Helianthus* refers to the sun, and these are sun loving plants. They can grow six to ten feet tall! The flowers do have the appearance of suns. In a field of Sunflowers there they are... hundreds of little suns all turning their faces in unison to catch the sunlight. The flower petals are a yellow orange color and surround a flat disk filled with seeds. If you are timely you can harvest most of the seed heads before the goldfinches do. I always leave seed heads for them to harvest so they will have food for the winter too.

The seeds are high in nutrition and easy to remove when they are ripe. The Sunflower has alternate, rough, hairy leaves, up to twelve inches in length. The roots of the plant go deep into the soil and leach out many minerals as they grow.

People have known about Sunflowers for a long time. Sunflower seeds have been found by archeologists in containers dated at three thousand years old.

What if your food was also medicine? Somehow our bodies know this is the truth of things. Roasted Sunflower seeds contain phosphorus, calcium, iron, trace copper (which helps the body utilize iron), iodine, fluorine, potassium, and magnesium. This is good rich food, rich in minerals the body needs, and in the amounts needed.

My Grandmother would hang the heads to finish drying in late summer (she had the most interesting kitchen rafters!). Sometimes she would save the seeds for snacks. But often times she would grind the seeds (hand grinder) and put them in a pot with water. The seed casings would float and she would skim them off. When the shells were gone she simmered the seeds until the oil floated to the surface of the kettle. This oil she used for nutritious baking. The remaining seeds she would roast and grind into flour. She could really cook!

Sunflower leaves can be dried and kept as medicine for intermittent fevers. This is the kind of fever for which quinine was used. Sunflower leaves are good gentle medicine for whatever illness causes the fever.

As surely as there are many different mints in the Mint Family, so there are different sunflowers in the Sunflower family. The plant called by the strange common name of Jerusalem Artichoke is actually a Sunflower. There is no doubt when you see the flower. The yellow central disk is surrounded by ten to twenty yellow petals. It is perennial, with thick, oval toothed, opposite leaf whorls. The stem is thick and hairy and the roots go deep to enrich the plant with ground minerals.

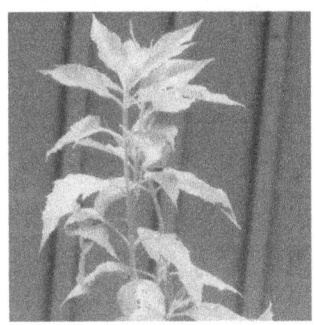

FIELDS
Helianthus tuberosus

Jerusalem Artichoke

The part of the **Jerusalem Artichoke** harvested for food and medicine is the root tuber. The root looks like a small potato. This tuber contains inulin, which is a helpful starchy substance. The tuber can be peeled, sliced and eaten raw, and is much like a water chestnut in texture. Or the tuber can be cooked and added to soups or stews, very tasty.

It is good to dig up and move the bed of Jerusalem Artichokes about every three years. They need the mineral abundance of a fresh place to grow, and they cannot move on their own. We can, indeed, have a relationship with plants. The root tubers are plentiful. Some are food for people, and some can be divided and planted like seed potatoes in a new place for the plant to grow. Wait until after the first frost to dig the tubers, as it is their time of greatest food energy, for their own future generations and as the gift of food for People.

My grandmother ate many of the tubers, as the starch was not a problem for her diabetes. She also gathered the seeds of this plant as a medicine. For rheumatism or arthritis, she simmered a quarter cup of raw seeds in a quart of water. She cooked the seeds until the liquid was reduced by about one fourth. When the seeds were filtered out, my grandmother added a heaping tablespoon of honey to the liquid, then kept the mixture in the refrigerator, one tablespoon a day for aches and pains.

There are many good things to eat growing comfortably in fields near us. Uncooked vegetables carry the richness of the Earth undiluted by being cooked into submission. Sunflowers are easy to grow, and the birds will gladly eat whatever seeds you miss.

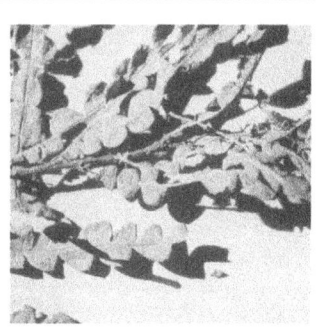

FIELDS
Comptonia peregrina

Sweet Fern

My herb mother called this plant *Myrica asplenifolia*, although its common name, **Sweet Fern**, does describe the leaf shape. The leaves of this plant resemble those of the spleenwort fern called Asplenium. Sweet Fern is an aromatic, deciduous (looses leaves annually) shrub that grows in the open sandy meadows of northern Wisconsin. It forms colonies, or sometimes entire fields of bushes about three feet tall. The fern-like leaves have yellowish resin dots which make them a fragrant plant donor for Kinnikinnik.

The bushes have burr-like flowers in April and May, depending on the weather for the when of things. Actually, the male flowers are catkins clustered at the tips of the branches. The female flowers are the bur-like clusters that grow below the catkins on the Sweet Fern bush. The plant lets the winds of Spring take care of pollination.

This is the first herbal tea I ever sampled. My herb mother made Sweet Fern and Rose petal tea, and it tasted wonderful. I, therefore, thought that herbal teas were marvellous. Well, sampling some of the earthier blends have modified this first decision. Though I have never doubted that plant infusions would do their part in a healing.

Sweet Fern happily grows in the same neighborhood with Jack Pine Trees. The Sweet Fern roots have nodules that fix nitrogen in the soil. They make the field a richer and more attractive breeding ground for themselves. Sometimes they will crowd out some of the softer plants. The leaves stay on the plants over winter and deer find this a welcome food as the snow gets deeper.

An infusion of Sweet Fern leaves is good for fever, stomach cramps, and diarrhea. It is mild and gentle, and a good choice for children. If the leaves are infused for several hours, the tea water is good for skin problems or mysterious rashes.

The People gathered Sweet Fern leaves to line their birchbark makuks before gathering Blueberries. The Native People called this plant Gibaime Nunagwus, which means Cover Blueberries. Berries covered with Sweet Fern leaves would not mold. The same fresh leaves were also used to keep winter clothing and blankets sweet smelling and free of mold. This plant is a good friend winter or summer.

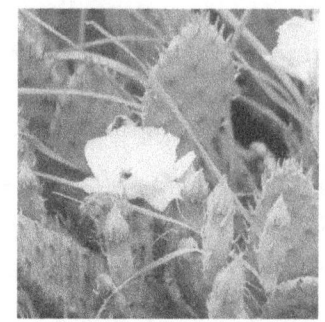

FIELDS
Opuntia humifusa

Prickly Pear Cactus

About halfway up the state of Wisconsin there is an end to the rich glacier fed loamy soil and the sand country begins. Wisconsin sand was provided by time and erosion from the many sedimentary rock formations. It is delightful if seemingly contradictory to find Cactus growing here. But **Prickly Pear** grows happily all across the central part of North America, from Texas to Minnesota.

Prickly Pear grows to about twelve inches tall. It has jointed pads with tufts of sharp bristles. The thick covering on the pads helps conserve water inside the plant. The bristles easily turn away animals that might try to browse on the juicy pads. Early in the summer the Cactus pads produce largy, showy yellow flowers followed by oval fruit cases. I had heard these fruits were good to eat so I picked one and put it in my shirt pocket to taste later. It wasn't long before I realized the fruit also has tiny bristle spines that poked right through my shirt. It tasted a little like cucumber, but I decided I wasn't hungry enough to gather food from such a bristly plant!

The Cactus pads can be peeled (carefully), and used as a poultice for cuts and puncture wounds. There must be some anti-bacterial activity since the inside tissue of the Cactus pads can also be steeped as a tea and used for lung problems.

I suspect Prickly Pear is tonic for the body in its attempts to regulate the PH level in the body. If the PH is too acidic the body needs help with the mineral imbalance which is a part of certain conditions. This Cactus appears to be of help for rheumatism, gout, and the tendency toward kidney stones.

This is a plant I would like to research further if I can find enough growing to allow for careful gathering. Sometimes I have to wait until the Spirit of the Plant says it is willing to share its medicine with the People. Even though I do not always gather Plants, I can still wonder about these things.

WOODS

On our walk we have reached the end of the open field. Along the edge of the field the place of trees begins. This is a noticeably different place. There is shade from the trees and less light comes down unfiltered. Plants are very clever beings; they have found ways to adapt to the change, in fact many of the smaller plants cannot survive in full sunlight. The outer edge of the woods is its own world. It is unique. Part of the day it has sun, part of the day it has shade. The most obvious residents are the raspberries, as they love the edges. If raspberries get full sun the berries dry up too fast. If they have full shade the plant cannot capture enough sun energy to put out an abundant crop of berries. They need edges!

Okay, edges are also a bit formidable; Grape vines, Sunflowers, and Nettles like them. We will find a path rather than thrash our way through the "edge" plants. And strangely, once we are fully into the woods there are not that many plants growing under the trees.

The trees have grown tall keeping company with their own kind or with other trees who need the same kinds of growing conditions and soil composition. These "tall plants," the trees, are a wonder to behold. We are walking in a woods that planted itself. There is variety! This is a good way for the forest. If an insect pest infects one kind of tree, we do not lose all the trees.

The air is different here; it is cooler and there seems to be more moisture in the air, a lot more moisture. Trees breathe, as do all plants. This breathing is just more noticeable in the woods. The plant kingdom and the animal kingdom are in balance; the animals breathe in oxygen and breathe out carbon dioxide, the plants breathe in the carbon dioxide and give off oxygen. The balance continues in the gifting of food to the animals by the plants. The animals in return leave rich mineral fertilizer on the forest floor, which is returned to the plants for their life cycle.

How can I talk about animals in a plant book? My only justification is that trees and plants often utilize these "moving seed dispersal units" to travel. Sometimes the seeds stick to animal fur, sometimes the seeds go all the way through the digestive tract of a browsing animal and reach the ground with their own fertilizer at the ready. Plants and animals are much older beings than we are and have figured these things out. We are the newcomers to the Earth.

I will pause for just a moment longer to talk about the way of deer. A deer can move through the woods without making a sound (I don't know how they do this with four legs to manage). Deer do not hibernate, they stay awake all winter. Their hair is hollow so that it is an "insulated" covering, and very warm. I have seen deer sit down on their back haunches and slide down a snow covered hill like a toboggan! The other marvel I have observed is their curiosity. I have seen them walk out on a pier, overlooking a river, and just stand there looking left and right. They are unbelievably curious. Of course, many people say only humans are intelligent, but I've come to know better.

Moving back to plants, I would like to share with you an explanation of why the leaves change color, this is the way my grandmother explained it—the leaves change color to remind us of what the tree contains, in case someone forgot.

If the leaves turn yellow there is no strong acid in the tree. Some trees don't turn color at all. After a frost the leaves just turn brown. The brown comes from the tannin in the tree. Like the Elm tree, whose leaves are yellow for a day, then the next day brown along the leaf edges, and next the whole leaf is brown. The oaks have a red color for a short time then turn brown. If a tree makes both yellow and red pigments then the leaves turn orange.

If the leaves turn red there is sugar in the tree. If the red leaves change to brown then the tannin is much stronger than the sugar, as with oaks. When the leaves stay red it means there is sugar in the tree and we can get it out. Most Maple species are good for making sugar. We could also tap a Birch or a Box Elder. Each of these trees turns a different shade of red. The more sugar the redder they get! The sugar trapped in the leaves gets heated during the warm time of the day. At night the cold turns the sugar solid.

As autumn approaches the tree realizes it is time to withdraw its lifeblood, otherwise when the frost comes it would freeze. The tree withdraws the chlorophyll which appears green in the leaves. Actually chlorophyll is blue, it appears green because it combines with the yellow pigment. When the chlorophyll is pulled back into the tree the other pigments are left behind in the leaves. Sometimes a leaf will have traces of green pigment along its ribs. When the tree called back the chlorophyll some got stuck and didn't return to the tree. Little cork plugs form where the leaf attaches to the stem. That is why in autumn you hardly have to touch a leaf and it snaps off the branch!

This is only one aspect of the life cycle of trees. These are wonderful tall beings, and each tree has its own life story. I am grateful for the medicinal sharing and the shaded beauty which is also a gift of the trees.

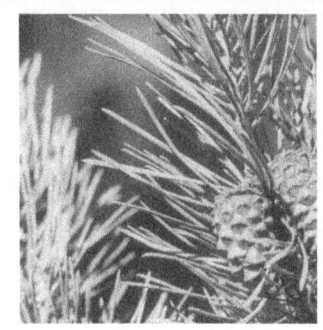

WOODS
Pinus banksiana

Jack Pine

Jack Pine is a small, scruffy looking evergreen, it really looks like a bad hair day tree! This little pine grows happily in the sunlight of a savannah, which is a sandy prairie with trees in it. The needles grow in pairs, about an inch long, and they are curved and twisted. Probably the most distinctive feature of Jack Pine are the reflexive (curved back on themselves) cones. These gray, resin covered cones may stay on the tree for years. As the tree gets taller the lower branches die off, adding to the unkempt appearance of this tree.

It sounds like I don't like this tree, but I do. I have photographed these gnarly little cones many times. One of the warblers, the Kirtland Warbler, will only nest in a Jack Pine tree. The bird, and the tree which is not considered a "valuable lumber tree," thrives in the state managed areas of the Michigan forest.

Part of the difficulty for Jack Pine is that it usually needs fire for its seeds to germinate. The fire burns the resin coating off the cones so the seeds are released. This little Pine becomes one of the first colonizers after a fire. I suppose this is why the tree does well in a savannah setting. The dry grasses burn easily and quickly, and give Jack Pines an opportunity to introduce their children to a renewed field.

The roots of this tree are long, white, and flexible. They can be split easily and the Native Americans used these roots for strong lashing, like the support frame of a wigwam. The pitch of Jack Pine is antiseptic (and a bit sticky). Dissolving the pitch in boiling water makes a good inhalant for congestion. I am old enough to remember when inhalants were commonly used for coughs. Breathing in medicated vapors, which is what vaporizers do, is a very direct method to get the medication where it needs to go.

Trees live for many years. They become a place of food and shelter for other creatures. Ruffed grouse and spruce grouse stay in the Northlands for the winter. For these hardy birds the Jack Pine is home, and provides a tasty meal of needles whenever food is needed.

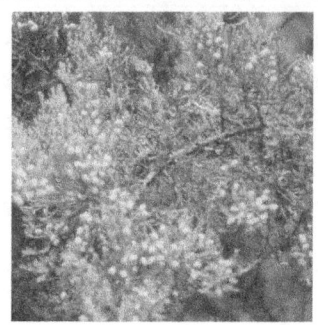

WOODS
Juniperus virginiana

Red Cedar

This is a slow growing evergreen that prefers sandy areas. It is drought resistant and lives up to three hundred years. **Red Cedar** grows about forty feet tall. It has thin, fibrous, reddish-brown bark which makes the Red Cedar very susceptible to fire, the bark burns easily.

The needles are sharp and prickly (very different from soft White Cedar), they are about a quarter to a half inch in length. The branches of the Red Cedar begin growing low on the trunk and continue right up to the top of the tree. It makes a nice "ladder tree" for pre-flight young bluejays! I have seen them hop from branch to branch right back up to their nest.

Red Cedar produces a blue, berry-like fruit that stays on the tree all year long. The cedar waxwings really love these berries. They will line up along a branch and pass the berries beak to beak until all birds get something to eat.

The People used fragrant inner bark to make floor mats for wigwams. These mats resist mildew and hold up for quite a while. Yes, this is the wood used in the making of cedar boxes. Cedar boxes were, and are, used to store woolens and other cloth to defend it against moths. The Native Americans also used this wood to make dugout canoes, it is rather soft and easy to hollow out. The people of the Great Lakes usually made canoes of Birch bark. However, if a large Red Cedar offered itself, it could become a dugout canoe.

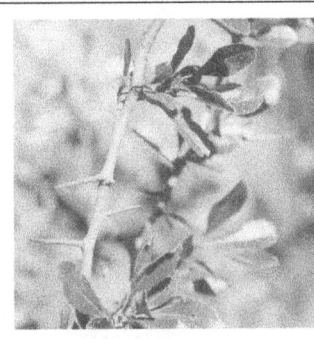

WOODS
Crataegus spp.

Hawthorn

This wide crowned, sun loving tree is a member of the Rose family, and the reason is apparent ... thorns! The Native people called it Minesagawunj, which means "Having Fruit and also Spikes." This tree is well defended from animal browsers. The Hawthorns (thornapples) form dense thickets of themselves, all about the same size. They very easily crowd out any other trees.

It is not easy to describe a Hawthorn tree because there are so many hybrids. They are the champions of evolution in the present age. In general the leaves are alternate. They are single, or double, toothed (and sometimes lobed). The twigs have thorns. The blossoms are usually whitish-pink, five petaled, with little or no fragrance. They are insect pollinated, and this works very well, and many blossoms become many thornapples.

The thornapples vary in size and sweetness. Some are sweet enough to eat as "little apples," but others are small, hard and bitter. As a youngster I would taste the thornapples. If they were good I ate them, but if they were bitter I used them as ammunition for my slingshot. I surely planted some trees with my target practice. The colors of the thornapples vary, too. Anything from yellow to red to black can be found. Sometimes the apples stay on the tree all winter.

It takes two years for the thornapples to germinate, so some just wait on the tree. The Hawthorns contain saponins, glycosides, flavonoids, ascorbic acid, and tannin.

These Hawthorn trees make excellent nesting sites for many bird species, like mourning doves, flycatchers, catbirds, and cardinals. The Shrike, a small predator bird, does not have grasping talons to hold its food. They catch their prey, then pin their food on a thorn for eating.

Medicinally the Hawthorns have much to offer. They are being researched and used as a tonic for the heart and circulation system. Hawthorn helps the heart find a normal, gentle beat (helps avoid palpitations). The Hawthorn leaves and flowers may be of help for congestive heart failure problems. This is a common difficulty for the elderly. An infusion or a tincture could be used. But if the condition is difficult, I would choose the tincture which is stronger and easier to measure for a dose.

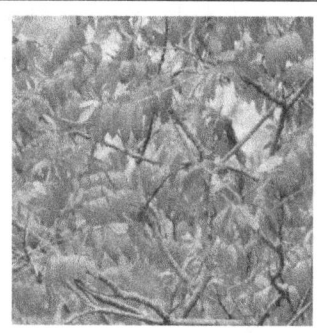

WOODS
Rhus typhina

Staghorn Sumac

Sumac is a small tree which sometimes appears to be a shrub. It grows about fifteen feet at its tallest. Sumac enjoys making little colonies filling open areas with all male or all female clones of itself. Sumac has a relationship with gently sloping hillsides, as there is a certain angle just right for Sumac to grow. This particular angle often happens along roadsides, where you will notice Sumac groves. Perhaps you won't notice until the fall of the year when the Sumac bursts into a reddish-burgundy blaze of color. Sumac is one of the first to announce the changing of the seasons.

The leaves are alternate and compound. There are ten to twenty lance shaped leaflets that are shiny green on top and whitish underneath. The Sumac twigs are covered with soft hairs as are the cone-shaped red fruit clusters that form at the top of the trees. These fruits are good food for pheasants, grouse, turkeys, crows, and cardinals. I wonder if perhaps the cardinal chose to be red so that he won't be seen eating Sumac berries at the top of the tree. Different birds are comfortable in different zones of a tree. The robins sit in the lower third of a tree, the bluejays like the middle area, and cardinals and little tiny warblers like the view from the top.

Rhus glabra, or Smooth Sumac, is the second most common Sumac species. It is called "smooth" because the twigs do not have the fine hairs and the fruits are less fuzzy. Both sumac species have rather straight trunks and branches. The center of the branches is a soft, pithy region which is easy to remove. The Native People used the branches of this tree to make pipe stems. The outer wood is easily shaped and forms a shiny coating, like lacquer, when it is rubbed with a cloth.

Both Sumac trees have medicinal gifts to share. The red berries can be dried for winter use to make a lemony flavored tea high in Vitamin C. Sumac leaf tea is a helpful tonic for borderline diabetics and those with chronic asthma. The inner bark of the sumac is actively antiseptic and helps stop bleeding. This inner bark can be pounded then mixed with a lotion to help prevent infection in a cut. We humans have a flair for punching holes in our outer skin covering, so it is good to have trees to help with our clumsiness.

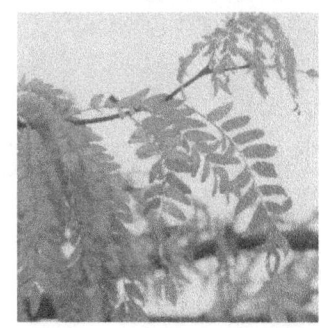

WOODS
Robinia pseudoacacia

Black Locust

The **Black Locust** grows to about fifty feet tall. This is a fast growing tree which only lives about one hundred years. It seems there is a relationship between being fast growing and being short-lived. Perhaps the tree puts a lot of "life energy" into the growing tall process and the cost is paid in shorter time of life in this cycle.

Locust is unusual in appearance; the main trunk is usually twisted or crooked. The bark is dark reddish-brown, thick, coarse and deeply furrowed. This is not a pretty tree, but it is rich in character. This particular tree does not have any relationship with People, but this is by the choice of the People! The twigs have short pairs of sharp prickles at the base of the leaf stalks. The leaves are compound with about sixteen small, smooth edged leaflets all wearing serious armament which discourages "people-animals" who have no protective fur covering. At dusk or during rain the leaflets curl and droop. This is the "acacia behavior" that earned the Locust its Latin name.

The flowers are insect pollinated. Butterflies have no trouble working with this tree and are given rich pollen for their efforts. The butterflies try to help but the main strategy for reproduction in Black Locust is cloning. The Black Locust occurs in thickets, impassable thickets! The roots of the "mother tree" sprout in the area nearby. Suddenly there is a place of shelter for rabbits and quail to hide from predators.

This tree is in the pea family, and has the root nodules that fix nitrogen in the soil. Locust may begin in eroded limestone places, but it helps build a richer soil for other trees who will be able to thrive after the shorter life cycle of the Locusts has ended. The short, flat, brown seed pods stay on the tree through the winter. Locust provides shelter and food for those animals who stay awake through the winter.

This Locust has character. It waits to leaf out in Spring until after most other trees have already done their "leafing." It waits in the field looking like a skeleton until its time to bloom. Where this tree grows you will not find Goldenrod growing. The two species do not grow together (allelopathic). Each plant produces chemicals which make life difficult for the other to thrive. I do not know why these two beings are in disagreement, but I suspect they do.

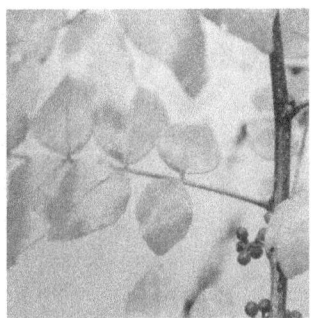

WOODS
Zanthoxylum americanum

Prickly Ash

Along the banks of rivers, or where the woods have just begun, is where you'll find thickets of **Prickly Ash**. These are even more formidable than the Black Locust. The thorns are paired and grow along all the branches. What is most noticeable is that there are many, many stems! Prickly Ash is actually a very tall shrub, up to fifteen feet tall. It creates a protective area for many animals.

The leaves are compound with seven to eleven oval leaflets. The leaves and the stems are covered with glandular dots, making this plant very aromatic. The flowers are small, green, tight clusters that mature into tiny quarter inch brown pods. Each pod has two tiny black seeds. I have been turned aside by a thicket of Prickly Ash that has allowed a deer to enter at full speed. Still I ask this tree to share its medicine. It is worth the risk, just like the sweetest of Raspberries which grow on canes so prickly they can rip denim!

The fragrant bark of the Prickly Ash is what contains the medicine. I suspect part of the gift comes from the small resin dots. In an emergency the bark can be chewed as treatment for toothache, as it has the same numbing effect as cloves. Otherwise, gather the bark during the active springtime. The trees draw up fluids in the barometric abundance of early spring, just like the Maple trees do. It is a phenomenon even humans can feel (we call it spring fever).

A tea made from the bark stimulates digestion. Prickly Ash tea moves the entire digestive tract into a quicker rhythm. Sometimes digestion gets so lethargic that food can ferment in the intestines. The tea also stimulates the lymph system and is a diaphoretic to help the body sweat out toxins.

There is even more stimulation in the Prickly Ash tea. The circulation of the blood is also stimulated, especially in the legs. Prickly Ash tea is very helpful for varicose veins, leg cramps, and certain kinds of chronic arthritis and rheumatism. I keep some Prickly Ash bark on hand for the circulation problems, it is very helpful for our "elders." To find safe, helpful medicine is worth a few scratches, so always carry a pair of leather gloves in your gathering pack.

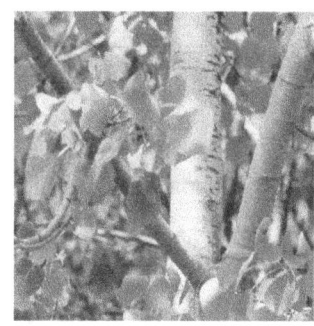

WOODS
Populus tremuloides

Quaking Aspen

This is the **Quaking Aspen**, a member of the Willow family, and it has the flexibility to dance in the wind. Trees have a deep relationship with the wind; from pollination, which leads to the life of future generations of a tree being, to the glory of moving in dance with the energy of the wind.

Aspen can grow in most any kind of soil. They range from Canada to Mexico. This is a pioneer species. When an area has burned or been lumbered off, one of the first trees to resettle the area are the Aspens. They keep company with Balsam Fir and Jack Pine watching over fields of Sweet Fern and Bracken Fern, which live in the barren soil of a disturbed area. Aspen loves the sunlight, and its leaves are beautiful in the summer light. The root clones grow to the surface and create thickets of Aspen with its oldest tree at the center of the Aspen island.

The Aspen puts out its flowers before the leaves come out on the branches. The male flowers are on one tree, the female on another. Without leaves, there is no interference with pollination. Almost everyone eats Aspen. The animals line up to munch according to their needs. Beaver will claim he "loves Aspen the most." The insects are a close second, with over three hundred insects that eat Aspen! Old Aspens with wide trunks often provide a home for the Hairy Woodpecker. The woodpecker digs a den in the soft wood, and its young eat some of the insects that eat the Aspen.

The Aspen leaves are almost round with a small point at the tip. The leaf stem is flattened and very flexible; it moves easily. Aspen bark is early springtime food for porcupines and black bears. Beaver takes the entire tree for lodge building and winter food. In winter the Aspen branches feed deer, elk, moose, and those long-legged snowshoe hares. The Aspens will populate an area until they are shaded out by the taller species of trees which are part of a mature, or "climax" forest.

People also depend on the Aspen for medicine. There is salicin, an aspirin like compound in the bark. The bark is also a hemostat for cuts, as it helps close the wound and lessen the pain. At the end of long winters, the cambium bark was emergency food for a starving People.

WOODS
Corylus cornuta

Beaked Hazelnut

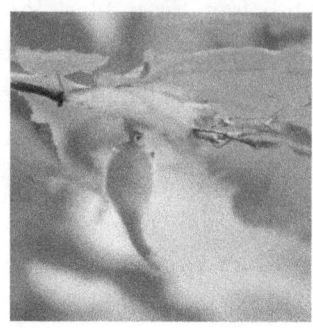

Hazelnuts grow at the edges of the woods. They are a shrub-tree growing up to twelve feet tall. Hazelnut belongs to the Birch Family. This is most noticeable in Spring when the catkins form near the tiny red female flowers. Since the leaves have not come out, the wind can easily help with the ongoing of the Hazelnuts. Leaving nothing to chance, this tree also forms root clones, so there is not just one Hazelnut in an area.

The leaves are double-toothed, alternate and oval in shape, and grow on long, stout twigs. The nuts that form are hairy with ragged husks. The end of the nut is elongated and looks a little like the beak of a bird. They grow in clusters of two to four nuts. The Hazelnut has a relationship with chipmunks. Late in the summer, on a certain day (perhaps the chipmunks can smell the ripeness), the Hazelnut trees are filled with squadrons of chipmunks. They chew around the nuts and drop them to the ground. The chipmunks fill their cheek pouches with fallen nuts and run off with them. I think the tree allows this because as with other "squirrel people" some of the buried nuts are forgotten and become nicely planted Hazelnut trees.

I gather as many Hazelnuts as I may need on the day the chipmunks designate. Do not gather where the chipmunks are, as they will drop nuts on your head. The Hazelnut is in the same Genus as the American Filbert. This is a tasty nut that can be eaten raw or roasted. Before there were flour mills, the People would roast the Hazelnuts and grind them for flour. These nuts have twenty-five percent protein, fifteen percent carbohydrate, and sixty percent fat.

For a People who lived outside over difficult winters, this kind of food energy was essential.

This is one of the first trees my herb mother talked about. She trimmed a Hazelnut twig piece into a short stick whittling a toothpick at one end and a toothbrush cluster of bark on the other, and then began brushing her teeth with the bristly end. She asked if I thought that Native Americans never brushed their teeth! My herb mother also told me a Hazelnut bark poultice was a good treatment for skin cancer sores which are caused by too much sunlight on the skin. The People did not have the word "cancer," but the sores have been a problem for people a long time. I wonder if we did the right thing genetically to give up a protective covering of fur.

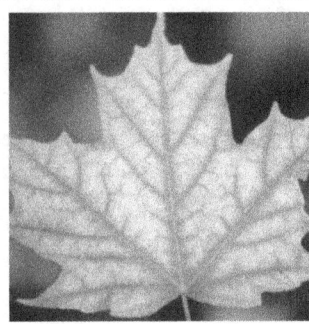

WOODS
Acer saccharum

Sugar Maple

Little Brother, Maumee (field mouse), where have you found food during this long, difficult winter? This was the question asked of the tiny mouse who first tasted the sap of a **Maple** tree. The People call this tree Aninaatig which means, our good tree. The sap of the Maple is cooked down to sugar every March. It can be stored easily and its high energy food is there for the People all through the year. The anthropologists refer to this kind of activity as, "primary forest efficiency." The People lived year round in the forests of the Great Lakes area, and the trees were neighbors and friends. There were no supermarkets, all that was needed came directly from the Earth. That is still true today, we just don't notice. Now we work for money to give to someone who works with the abundance of the Earth to provide food for us.

The Maple trees are still there, growing tall in the woods. Maple has opposite branches, while most trees have alternate branches. The outer bark has chevron markings very much like the markings found on Birch tree bark. You can probably find fallen leaves under the "winter Maple" to help you decide what tree you are looking at. Maples are shade tolerant, and they live up to three hundred years. The Maples prefer the rich lime soil of the Great Lakes area. These trees are insect pollinated and have an abundant seed crop about every four years. Maples fill the woods with their children. Only two things can interfere with the life cycle of the Maples, warm temperatures and pollution. Maples like to breathe cool, clean air.

When the days of early Spring bring temperatures of about forty degrees in the daytime, and twenty degrees at night, the sap begins to rise in the trees. This is a barometric mystery that gives the birds a reason to sing! As dignified people we pretend we do not experience this. We have inner fluids that also experience the seasonal changes.

It takes about forty gallons of tree sap to yield one gallon of Maple syrup. That's a lot of cooking! The taste of real Maple syrup is like nothing else on Earth. Early Spring is a wonderful time to be out in the hardwood forests. The hawks are in courtship. The Canada Geese and Sandhill Cranes are coming back for the Summer season. The sky is filled with song, you'll like it.

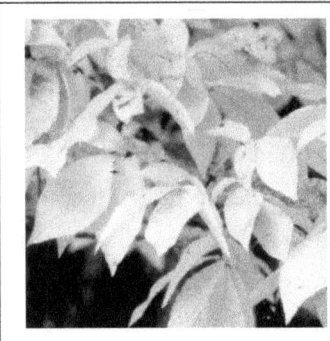

WOODS
Carya ovata

Shagbark Hickory

In Autumn the squirrels will lead us to the **Hickory** trees. In a frenzy of gathering, these rascals gladly drop nuts on your head.

Hickory bark is loose, and grows in shaggy strips that look like old, gray, warped shingles. The leaves are alternate on the branches, and compound (more than one leaflet per leaf). There are usually five leaflets, the upper three are large. These are distinctive leaves; the widest part of the leaf is in the middle, and is tapered at both ends.

This tree is a fine "forest elder." Hickory doesn't flower until it is twenty years old. The nut crops begin at age forty! Hickory trees have an abundant nut production every third year. Perhaps they need the time to see how many young trees have sprouted from the accidental plantings of the squirrels. It sounds kind of funny, but the Hickory trees need the squirrel activity for reproduction as much as the smaller plants need the help of bees and butterflies.

Hickory is truly a hardwood tree. The People chose this wood for making bows; the heartwood at the outside of the bow, the sapwood facing the archer. The bowstring came from sinew which occurs naturally along the back of a deer. Whether Plant or Animal, nothing is wasted, that is part of the balance of life, whether we realize it or not.

Hickory makes the warmest firewood. Many branches fall to the forest floor by the action of the wind. The People found it there for the gathering, while the trees continued to grow and make more branches, and delicious nuts.

If you have tried to get Hickory nuts out of the shells you know there must be a trick to it, and much work! The People would put the nuts into a low fire to roast. After the roast they smashed the nuts with a rock and put the results into a kettle of water. The shells floated and could then be skimmed off. The nut meats could be dried at this point, or cooked to yield the oil first, then dried. Nut oil is high energy food, very important for a physically active People.

The People did not grow Wheat, they grew Corn which could be ground into flour to make bread. In autumn the People moved from place to place to harvest nuts and seeds. With store bought food the seeds and nuts are there for the animals, if we only let the trees grow!

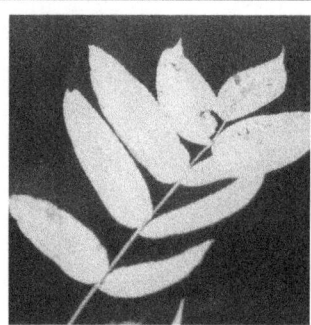

WOODS
Juglans cinerea

Butternut
(White Walnut)

Butternut is a short tree, about fifty feet tall, with wide spreading branches. The leaflets are opposite, finely toothed and somewhat rounded at the base. The easiest way to tell White Walnut from Black Walnut is by the tip of the leaflet branch. If the leaflet tip has a single leaflet at the end, then it is the White Walnut. With Black Walnut the leaflet ends with a pair of leaves.

Butternut likes moist forests, lowlands or dry limestone soil. It does not form colonies, but rather mixes in with other trees in the area, including Black Walnut trees. The husk is shaped like a lime with a greenish-brown color. This lime shell is hairy and sticky. There are ridges of reinforcement, so this is literally a tough nut to crack.

The catkins (slender branches of male flowers) form at the same time as the female flowers near the ends of the branches. They wait for the wind to do the pollinating. Butternut is a fast growing, short-lived tree with deep roots, well adapted to a cool climate. Butternut is a late bloomer; the leaves come out on the tree very late in spring and are dropped early in the fall. By mid Autumn the Butternut looks like a skeleton tree with only a generous supply of Butternuts lying underneath on the ground to give away its identity. Impatient pruners have cut down living trees not knowing how late a start this tree can have in spring.

The leaves and twigs have an aromatic sap and a soft covering of fuzzy hairs. The sap contains juglone, a plant chemical, which protects the area around the tree from other plants. The fallen leaves and twigs release their chemical into the soil providing a clear growth zone for the Butternut tree. Unfortunately, this does not protect the tree from a canker produced by a sac fungus. Eventually the entire tree is affected and slowly dies. This is a serious disease and the number of Butternut trees is diminishing.

In the past, when the Butternut trees were abundant, the Native People would gather the nuts and coax them out of the shells. The nuts were cooked down into a rich, buttery consistency. This was high calorie food that brought energy and good flavor to the People. The nuts were also chopped and cooked with venison stew to add a little fat to the protein of the meat. The time for gathering Butternuts is early in October. I have done this, and though it is a lot of work, the nuts are very good.

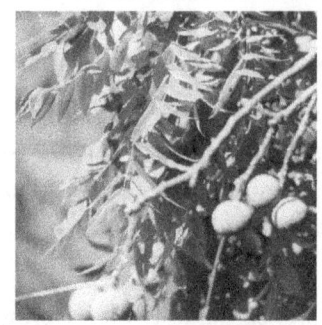

WOODS
Juglans nigra

Black Walnut

The **Black Walnut** tree also waits until late spring to leaf out. Before this happens the tree looks like a black furrowed skeleton with heavy branches in a zigzag pattern. Why? Black Walnut loves sunlight, and needs the light to grow and produce food. By zigging the branches there is maximum opportunity to catch sunlight even if other trees happen to grow nearby (clever tree). The Black Walnut also secretes the quinone compound juglone in large amounts from its bark, roots, and nut casings. This compound inhibits the growth of many other plants and trees, but it also inhibits the growth of its own seedlings! Hopefully a helpful squirrel will carry the nuts far enough from the parent tree to see to the future.

Squirrels are very helpful to the nut trees. They carry off the nuts to bury for another time and then forget just where it was they put all the nuts! Since it takes a full year of freeze and thaw to germinate the nuts, it is actually helpful if the squirrel chews on the nut casing. Those squirrel bites actually help the process by allowing moisture to seep into the shell. The rodents, with their sharp teeth have an easier time getting to the nut meats than we humans. We usually have to resort to a hammer or a nutcracker.

This Walnut also has compound leaves with about twenty leaflets per leaf. Remember this is the tree with two leaflets beside each other at the tip of the leaf. The bark is a dark, rich chocolate brown color and the nuts sometimes stay on the tree over winter to help you with identification. The leaves are finely toothed and have a spicy aromatic smell. Black Walnut does not like acidic soil, and it actually contributes to the alkalinity of the soil around itself. This tree shares space with Black Raspberries and the Wild Mints, so there must be some advantage for these plants in the relationship. Perhaps it is the less acidic soil they find attractive.

The leaves of Black Walnut have a medicinal sharing, they are astringent and anti-fungal. Walnut leaf tea can help with diarrhea, and as an external wash will help with athletes foot. There is also a small amount of the "juglone" in the leaves. This has some anti-tumor activity and is slightly sedative.

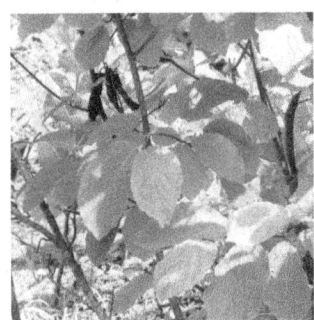

WOODS
Hammamelis virginiana

Witch Hazel

Witch Hazel is an understory shrub that fills in the area below the taller trees. It prefers dry wooded places. I have to call this a shrub because each clump of growth is an individual plant. This shrub grows up to fifteen feet tall and is tolerant of the shade in its growing place. Part of its plan to survive includes crooked stems that produce rather large oval leaves with scalloped edges. Having more leaf surface to work with lets the Witch Hazel make the most of whatever sunlight filters through the canopy.

Witch Hazel has its own unusual reproductive style. The little flowers come out in late autumn after the leaves have fallen. It is pollinated by tiny gnats who don't give up their foraging until the snow actually falls. The seed pods stay on the tree for a full year and utilize the time of flowering to pop open and propel their little black seeds up to twenty feet away from the parent tree! You can actually hear the pods when they open. The seed pods are protected from the winter freezing by a thick woody covering. They look like tiny wooden marbles hanging on little stems on the tree.

The Witch Hazel has a two-fold medicinal gift. First, I gather leaves to dry in the infamous brown paper bags. Then I gather some of the twigs at the ends of the branches. The twigs tincture out in water and alcohol to make a rubbing liniment. The alcohol I use is vodka so the tincture can be used internally or externally. As a massage liquid it is very good for sore muscles, especially in the legs. You probably know that light massage is good for people (it also feels good). Internally, this vodka tincture is a good mouthwash for bleeding gums. But if you buy Witch Hazel leaves the tincture will not be astringent and stop bleeding. In commercial products the tannins, which stop the bleeding, are leached out.

Store the dry leaves in a glass jar. These leaves can be crumbled for an infusion (tea) which when steeped for fifteen minutes, is helpful for internal bleeding of the lungs, stomach and hemorrhoids. People have had difficulty with hemorrhoids as long as there have been people. The Witch Hazel tea is also good for insect bites. Put a little liniment on the external place of the bite, then drink a cup of leaf tea to help the body deal with the insect venom. This is a very helpful shrub.

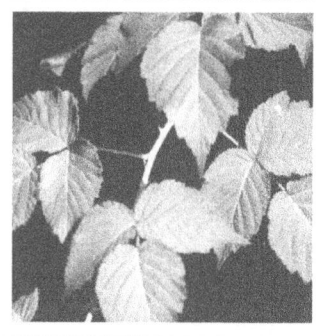

WOODS
Rubus species

Raspberry

At the edge of the woods there is a little shade. The **Raspberries** are not concerned we are here. They are well defended against our kind of animal! The stems are reddish canes with many erect thorns. This is a perennial, shrubby plant, and will be here for years to come.

Raspberry is a clever plant. The long canes lean over toward the open areas of the patch. When the ends of the canes reach the ground they become rooted to form a new Raspberry plant.

The bushes move slowly, but they do move, building fine, tangled, impenetrable areas of safety for animals who need protection from predators. I hope you are wearing a heavy, long sleeved shirt and, of course, your gloves.

We have come to gather some of the leaves. If the timing is right there may also be ripe berries where we can reach them. Many creatures eat the berries but seeds don't mind the journey through an animal, as they sprout from the animal droppings.

The berries contain fruit sugar, volatile oil, pectin, citric acid, malic acid, fragarine, and Vitamins A, B, C, and E. The berries, if we don't eat them all, can be tinctured with some of the leaves to make a mouthwash. The tincture is one half cup of water and one half cup of alcohol to cover about a half a cup of berries and crumbled leaves (dry leaves are better). Use a tightly sealed jar so you can shake it a couple times a day for two weeks. After you filter out the pulp through a clean cloth, add some water to dilute the mix.

Raspberry has a medicinal gift; it is astringent (stops bleeding), especially in the mouth. It helps with bleeding gums, canker sores, and sore throat. If it is too tangy for you, warm it up and add a little honey. Raspberry leaves also have a gifting for women. They are tonic to the uterus, and this only requires a tea made with the dry Raspberry leaves. Raspberry tea helps with cramps, regulates the cycle, and checks excessive bleeding.

I really believe the leaves of the "wild" Raspberry plants are a better medicinal. I don't know what genetic changes are involved in the "domesticated" Raspberry plants. I know the wild Raspberries taste sweeter to me, and I believe they are better as food and as medicine.

Gooseberry is a low shrub, maybe three feet tall. It has a spiny stem, lobed hairy leaves, and a green berry with white markings It is good to eat raw or cooked into jelly. Its cousin, the Smooth Gooseberry, is similar in appearance but with very few prickles, and therefore easier to harvest. The berry is also a little different in that it has a blue-black color. This fruit is high in Vitamin C and dries easily for winter storage.

A third Ribes bush, *Ribes americanum*, is called Black Currant as a common name. Its Ojibwa name is "Micidjiminagawunj," which means "fuzzy fruit." The berry is a furry black berry about the same size as the Gooseberries. The leaves of this shrub look a bit like Maple leaves and there are no thorns. This is the most medicinal of the Ribes. A tea made from the root bark was used to help the body produce more urine. Sounds strange, but that is how waste products are eliminated from the body. "Better out than in," especially with somewhat toxic waste products.

Unfortunately the "Ribes" are a host to something called blister rust which is a danger to Pine trees. Instead of planting Pine trees further from the places where the ribes grow, the entire genus is being eliminated. That kind of policy is not conservation, it is the genocide of the ribes. The medicinal gifts from these plants may be lost forever.

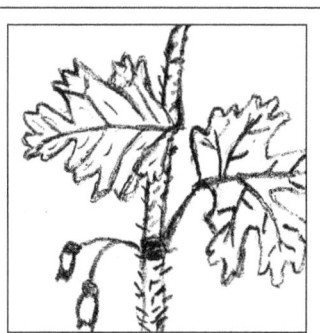

WOODS
Ribes species

Gooseberry

WOODS
Vitis species

Wild Grapes

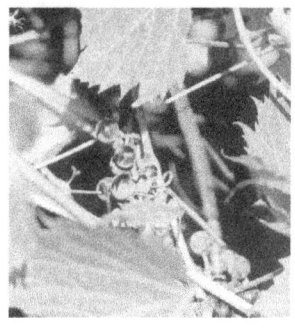

Grapes, belonging to the Genus *Vitis*, also have a blueish-black berry if they are allowed to grow. These wild Grapes are the genetic strength of so many Grape species. Plants clone easily and it is not difficult to come up with bigger and sweeter Grapes. Grape vines can grow very large. The Grape vine boosts its way up into the sunlight on the trunks of nearby trees, using tendrils that are actually modified flower stalks. This extra weight sometimes brings down trees which then opens up the forest canopy to the cycles of other kinds of plants.

Sometimes there are many Grapes, sometimes none. The Grapes may ferment on the vine, or dry to raisins, or be eaten by many hungry animals. Birds, and animals like the squirrel, raccoon, and bear all have a "relationship" with the fruit bushes. These are the seed carriers and tree planters who are fed and also see to the ongoing of the berry bushes.

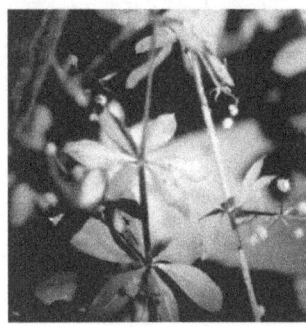

WOODS
Galium aparine

Cleavers

Cleavers stick to your clothing, to your dog, to everything. That's how they find new places to grow, the seeds just hitch a ride on anyone who passes by. If you walk into the Cleavers you probably won't need a gathering bag, you can harvest off your jeans. Cleavers have a long sticky clinging stem. The leaves grow in whorls along the stem. There are many species, so you will find little Cleavers and very large Cleavers.

I go out of my way to find and gather Cleavers, lots of them. They dry easily in the brown bag and crumble down for tea or capsules. The "above the ground" parts of the plant contain a glycoside called asperlosid, as well as gallotannic acid and citric acid. This plant has a powerful medicinal gifting for people. I don't think the plant medicine would work if we took it all apart in a lab and reduced it to its chemical components. Sometimes, I think it's most of the time, the plant needs to be there in its entirety to do its medicine. There are things in the plant that work together, and if some of these things are missing it just doesn't work. I believe many medicinal plants are written off scientifically because they won't come apart in the laboratory.

We will leave the plant intact and talk about what it can do. In general it is a diuretic and a kidney nudge. Okay, good, but what else? It is anti-inflammatory and anti-tumor. That's better, now we're getting somewhere. Most important for me is that Cleavers are tonic to the lymph system.

Cleavers are very effective for swollen glands, and work to promote lymph drainage. This is important with certain kinds of flu and colds that seem to get stuck in the lymph system. Most often I use this plant for women who have had surgery for breast cancer. Many times the surgery involves removing the lymph nodes under the armpits. This interferes with lymph circulation down the arm, and there is swelling in the wrist and hand. Cleavers share their medicinal action with this kind of condition. I can't think of anything more helpful to a cancer patient.

Cancer is difficult to work with. It is a "confusion" within the body, not caused by an outside agent (at least directly). Certain chemicals, or toxins, do seem to promote cancer growth, but in truth it is a loss of inner balance. There are many kinds of cancer and many plants willing to help the body restore balance.

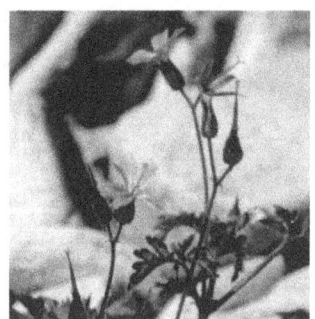

WOODS
Geranium maculatum

Cranesbill
(Wild Geranium)

This is a perennial plant which grows in the open woods or along the limestone beaches of the Great Lakes. This is my grandmother's Clan plant. She was Crane Clan; those who teach or lead, always remembering the history of the People. The plant got the common name **Cranesbill** from the beaked ovary of the plant. After the blossoming time, the ovary thickens and resembles the beak of a Crane!

In the woods this plant grows rather tall, with dark green palmately lobed leaves. The blossom is a white (sometimes pink) five petal flower. The stem is hairy and is usually purple in color. The growth pattern is rather bushy. When the plant grows along the shore it is different. There the plant is small, less than twelve inches tall, and the color of the entire plant is a lovely cranberry red. The stones along the shore are mostly white, so this plant is noticeably beautiful.

With Cranesbill the medicinal gift comes from the roots. This takes the life of the plant, so I only use this medicine for serious conditions. The root is astringent (stops bleeding), vulnerary (relieves pain and promotes healing), and anti-inflammatory. The powdered root will close open mouth sores. Cranesbill inhibits the growth of bacteria. I would not gather Cranesbill for that, since other plants will also do this.

It is the anti-hemorrhagic ability of this plant that sends me out to sing the "root gathering song." Add one tablespoon of dried root to a pint of cold water and simmer for about fifteen minutes This decoction is good for internal bleeding. Internal bleeding is a serious condition. You really can't get to it to put on a band aid, and surgery is always risky. It works best for this in combination with Marshmallow root or Slippery Elm bark, which form a protective covering of mucilage over the lining of the stomach to allow healing. People do bleed to death from internal injury. The gift of Cranesbill is the ability to treat this condition.

Herbalists today are often seen as the place of last resort. It is asking a lot of Plants to present only desperate, chronic, or critical conditions. When I ask the Plants about cancer they say, "why don't you ask before the person has cancer, or immune disorders, or arthritis?" Plants do their best healing by preventing a disease. Keep the body in the balance of good health, instead of trying to repair a lifetime of damage.

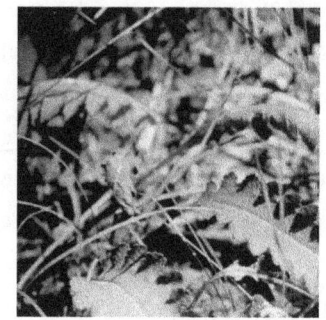

WOODS
Pedicularis canadensis

Wood Betony

Wood Betony looks like a Fern. The leaves are deeply lobed and they grow with the grace and flexibility of a Fern. There are no spores under the leaves and the flower makes it clear this is not a Fern! The yellow flowerlets on the terminal clusters are hooded like little yellow Snap Dragons. The pollen is rich, and the bees love this plant.

I gather the leaves, lots of leaves, but they are not easy to work with. The leaves are high in moisture, almost like a succulent plant. To dry, the leaves must be spread out on long sheets of paper towels. If the leaves touch each other they will mold, arggh! That is only the beginning of the challenge.

If the leaves get too much sunlight while drying they turn a strange grey-black color which is very embarrassing for an herbalist. People do not want to drink tea made from leaves that are blackened and look like cadavers, again, arggh. (The *growly* word after each sentence is my frustration as I learned about this plant.)

The most reliable drying method I have found has been the paper towel pathway, with another layer of paper towel over the top of the leaves so you can roll the entire package over, to dry the bottoms of the leaves. Some leaves jump out when you do this, but just pick them up and rearrange the leaves so they are not touching each other. Much patience is required.

Wood Betony also insists you hurry home from the gathering place to get the leaves spread out. They will only tolerate a couple hours of travel time, so don't gather any other plants while you are on a Betony hunt.

I put down a lot of Kinnik for this Plant, as it has been very patient while I learned its way. There are many leaves growing at the base of each plant, rather like Dandelion leaves. I only take a few leaves from each plant. Wood Betony forms colonies, so there are many of them in an area. I just crawl around until I have enough leaves. The Wood Betony grows under shade trees, a soft, comfortable place to spend some time in the summer.

This plant has a very important spiritual gift to share. A leaf infusion helps with the healing of nerve tissue, especially at the place of the synapses. One teaspoon per cup of boiling water at least twice a day helps with neck and back injuries. This is the only plant I know that is tonic to nerve tissue. It is worth all the bother to gather and dry.

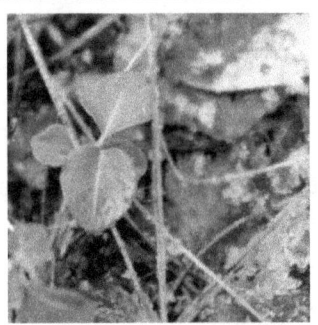

WOODS
Mitchella repens

Partridge Berry

FIELDS
Gaultheria procumbens

Wintergreen

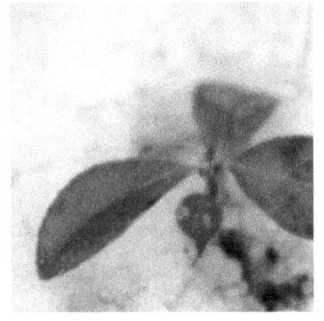

Partridge Berry is an evergreen plant. It stays green even under the snow. Partridge Berry has a trailing stem, and grows out over the ground into a mat or carpet of plant. The bright red berries are good food for Partridges, a hardy bird that spends the winter in the forests of the Great Lakes region. The People called this plant "Binemin" which means "Bird Berry."

Partridge Berry leaves are small, rounded, and grow opposite each other on the stem. The most distinctive feature is a yellow-white stripe down the center of each leaf.

My herb mother taught that shortly before the birth of a child the mother should eat fresh Partridge Berry plant. The green leaves and stems are lightly cooked and eaten as "greens." Something in the plant helps a woman's body prepare for the birthing process by toning the uterus and helping reduce pain. Partridge Berry was also used this way for young women with painful menstrual cramps. The medicinal gift is specific to the uterus.

Perhaps the Partridge Berry leaves could be steeped as a tea, but my herb mother preferred to have the young women eat the fresh plant. Either way is possible since the plant is there, year round, growing beneath the snow. In recent years I have not seen large patches of Partridge Berry growing in the forests, and it is a worry to me.

Wintergreen grows in the same environment with Partridge Berry. These plants are summer and winter neighbors. Both are perennial, and both are evergreen. Wintergreen only grows about three inches tall. The leaves are alternate, oval, and somewhat waxy in appearance. The leaves crowd the top of the stem, and just beneath them is the red Wintergreen berry. The leaves and especially the berry have a distinct fragrance and taste. They smell, and taste like "Wintergreen" (surprise).

Wintergreen tea tastes good and helps the body with the changing seasons. The People actually believed the changing of Seasons could affect the body causing aches and pains (so do I). Wintergreen contains methyl salicylate, so it helps prevent inflammation. It can be an inside-and-outside medicine. Drink a cup of the refreshing tea and let a Wintergreen massage oil soak into your aching joints.

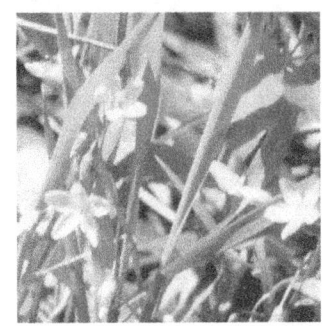

WOODS
Claytonia virginica

Spring Beauty

Spring Beauty has the right common name, as it is a beautiful little plant. It comes into flower in April but the flowers only last a few days. The blossoms are usually pale pink with darker iridescent pink stripes that lead a hungry insect right to the nectaries. The male and female flowers bloom at different times so there is no danger of self fertilization. The bee moves from a male flower on one plant to a female on another. It all works nicely for the plant.

The leaves of Spring Beauty are soft and slender, almost like blades of grass. The blossoms are light sensitive; they close at night or on dark cloudy days. Like this plant, bees also seem to need sunlight to warm themselves so they can fly in spite of their heavy bodies and transparent wings. When the seeds form, the plant has a device to eject the seeds away from the parent plant. Spring Beauty then spreads out into thickets.

There was a time when the tiny bulbs that produce these flowers were harvested by Native Americans in the early, very hungry days of spring. The bulbs are like tiny potatoes. Spring Beauty is not all that abundant, so I leave the bulbs for the mice and chipmunks who need food in early spring. The beauty of the plant is a lovely greeting on a warm April day, and that is enough for me.

At the same time, in the first days of spring, there are also blooming Hepatica flowers, Dutchman's Breeches, and the mottled leaf greenery of Trout Lilies. Sometimes there are still piles of unmelted snow in the woods! Why do these little plants risk the danger of frost? These plants, and some other early achievers, have discovered this is the time of sunlight in the thickly wooded places. Before the trees put out leaves the sunlight can reach the floor of the forest. Plants have good problem solving skills.

It is not surprising that trees and plants came to this planet many, years before people and other animals. The plants need only the energy of the sun and the dissolved minerals of the earth to survive. Okay, some rain, or handy subsurface water is also required, but it just amazes me that plants found a way to eat sunlight. There won't be a food shortage for them…although some day soon there may be a land shortage for any "wild plant" whose seeds are not sold in little packets.

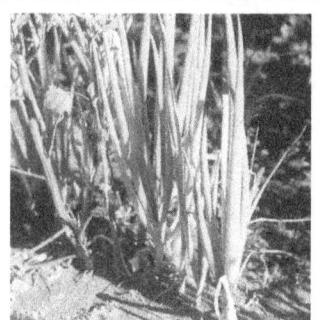

WOODS
Allium cernum

Wild Onion

WOODS
Allium tricoccum

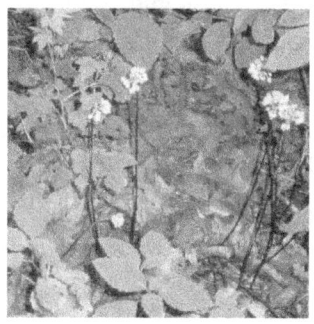

Wild Leek

Wild Onion is a perennial, and grows about twelve inches tall. The leaves are grass-like, and are soft and flat. The pinkish white flower forms a round cluster at the tip of an arching stem. My grandmother said the Indian word "Cicaga" was the name given to the city of Chicago because there were so many Onions there.

Like other Onions this Wild Onion is good to eat, just saute the bulbs and tender stems. If you simmer Wild Onions the tea helps with coughs, fever and even helps prevent the formation of kidney stones. Cutting and cooking the Onion releases the "allicin" from the Onion, which is antiseptic internally or externally.

Wild Leek is more common in the northern portions of the Great Lakes. This is the Allium species I am most familiar with. It is also a perennial growing about twelve inches tall. First the leaves come up from the ground. They are long and rather wide and have parallel veins. After the leaves turn yellow and wilt away, the flower stalk appears. It is a tall, slender, rounded stalk. The flower is a cluster of yellowish blossoms at the top of the stem. The Leek bulb is white and has fibrous roots at the lower end. I harvest Leeks carefully so intact bulbs are left in the patch to see to the future generations of Leeks.

Leeks like to grow in shady patches in a mature wooded area. They have been known to keep company with morel mushrooms. Both plants are worth finding and eating. There is a Potato Leek soup that will bring in hungry campers for a woodland dinner. However, my favorite use of Leeks is to melt butter and saute the chopped Leeks and then pour the butter over fresh popped popcorn. A bowl of popcorn and a campfire story is a wonderful way to spend an outdoor evening.

Like Onion, the Leek is also anti-bacterial and helps prevent colds. The raw Leek is also a good poultice for the pain of a bee sting. It is not difficult to find Leeks even without the leaves, as you will smell them along the trail.

The most medicinal of the "Alliums" is **garlic**, which sometimes escapes from gardens. Garlic lowers blood pressure and serum cholesterol. As a poultice it is anti-bacterial and anti-fungal. It even works on ringworm and athlete's foot. You can wash the smell off later, first kill the fungus.

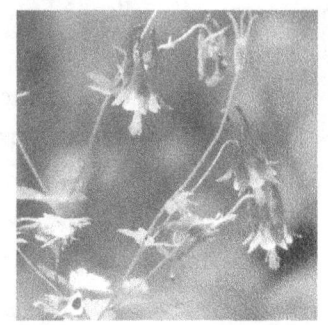

WOODS
Aquilegia canadensis

Columbine

Columbine is a perennial growing from a rhizome. It grows to about two feet tall and has alternate compound leaves divided into three lobes. Columbine loves the limestone soil of the Great Lakes region. It grows happily in the lightly wooded regions of conifers and deciduous trees who are adapted to the northern climate.

The most noticeable aspect of Columbine is the red flower (well, red on the outside and yellow on the inside). The flowers droop and have long nectar spurs. The spurs are the nectar repositories. They wait for the hummingbirds to do the pollinating with their long tongues. It is a perfect match of flower and bird. The long male stamins mature before the female pistils so there is no chance of self pollination. The willing hummingbird carries the pollen to another flower whose pistil is ready to accept the pollen.

It is a delight to watch the hummingbirds flit from one Columbine to the next. The nectar is sweet high energy food for the hummingbird. I have learned not to use a "man-made" hummingbird feeder. There are a number of reasons; one being the Columbine needs the help of the hummingbird to see to future generations. The second, and equally important reason, is artificial food can cause a visiting hummingbird to stay in the North too long in a summer season. The hummingbird needs to return South before the plants that normally provide food have stopped flowering. This way when the bird moves South there will still be flowers to feed on along the migration route. The hummingbird is programmed to time its journey to the cycles of the plants, and I do not want the little bird to starve on my account.

There is also a problem with fermenting sugar water in the plastic feeders, so I now only watch the birds feed on flowers.

If there are many Columbine flowers I will gather some of them to be a sweet, tasty garnish for a woodland salad. After the growing season when the seeds have dispersed on the wind, usually in fall, the rhizome forms a basal rosette of new leaves. These leaves stay green all through winter and give next summer's plants a head start on growing when the snow melts. This plant knows how short the summer can be in the North.

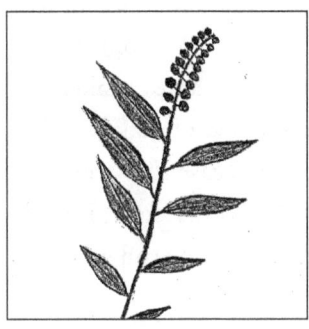

WOODS
Polygala senega

Seneca Snakeroot

Snakeroot grows about twelve inches tall from a thick rhizome. It is an interesting perennial, with alternate lance shaped leaves that do not have stalks. At the base of the plant stem the leaves are scales, and the entire stem is covered with glandular hairs. The flowers are small white pea shaped blossoms growing in a spike at the top of the stem.

In the fall of the year after the flowering is completed, it is time to gather some of the rhizome which holds the plant in the earth. This means some of the plants will offer up their life in this cycle, so I harvest carefully and sparingly. I put down Kinnikinnik and explain to the plant why I need the root. The seeds can be placed where the ground is open so there will be plants to replace what I have taken.

Seneca Snakeroot contains a trace of methyl salicylate which is helpful for rheumatism. We modern people pretend there is no such thing as rheumatism any more. But even if we now call it aches and pains in the muscles and tendons, it still hurts.

The root/rhizome can be tinctured in equal parts of alcohol and water, and mixes easily with other plants to make a cough syrup for pneumonia, pleurisy, asthma, and bronchitis. This plant may also be helpful for congestive heart failure. Congestive heart failure is not a heart attack, rather it is a buildup of fluid in the lungs and around the heart. If a person is active (not lying down all day) the body's circulation system clears this fluid. It is a common affliction for elders who are bed ridden.

The root could also be simmered in a water decoction but the saponins in the plant make the decoction foamy and suspicious looking. The medicinal action of Seneca Snakeroot is very powerful and should only be given in small doses (by the teaspoonful).

There are many plants with the common name "snakeroot." I think perhaps the colonists were very frightened of snakes and kept asking the Indians for some kind of remedy in case they were bitten. I am very fond of snakes, as they eat mice and other pests. I hope we can let them live and avoid future plagues spread by rodents.

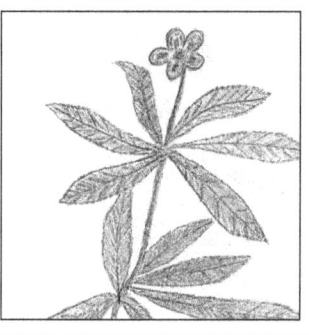

WOODS
Chimaphilia umbellata

Pipsissewa

Pipsissewa is a medicinal wonder and a delightful plant. I am glad it has held on to its Indian name. This is a perennial, growing up to twelve inches tall. Its Latin name, *Chimaphilia*, means "Winter Loving" and this plant is built to tolerate the doings of winter. It is an evergreen, growing happily under the snow cover if need be.

The leaves grow in whorls up the stem. Pipsissewa has waxy, toothed, and lanceolate leaves which are long, slender and pointed at the tip. They are shiny green on top and paler green underneath. Even the drooping white flowers at the top of the stem are waxy. Rain, snow, or sleet do not bother this plant. The blossoms mature into a brown capsule with many seeds. They are spread by the wind so you will find Pipsissewa growing in small groups rather than singly.

Medicinally Pipsissewa does a little of everything, and I have used it for a number of conditions. There was a time when the root of this plant was the only medicine for a condition called St. Vitus Dance. Fortunately, other medicines have been found to work with this condition and now I only gather leaves to use as medicine. You remember how to do this, only take a few leaves from each plant after offering Kinnik, then the plants can recover and be there if they are needed in the future. Pipsissewa and other medicine plants do things that have nothing to do with People. It is good to allow plants to live out their own purpose.

Pipsissewa contains arbutin (blood thinner), sitosterol, ursolic acid (cox two inhibitor), chimaphilin (anti-yeast), as well as resin, lignin, gum and saline substances. This means it is diuretic, antiseptic, astringent, and tonic to the kidneys and urinary system. A plant medicine that can help with yeast infections such as Candida which can become systemic is good medicine. As a tea (one tsp plant per cup of water) it helps with pain relief, backache, bladder infections, kidney stones, and the arthritic conditions caused by a buildup of uric acid in the body.

For complex conditions such as kidney stones, you might want to add some other plants to help with the condition (like Joe Pye Root). It is much easier to work with conditions like this before they send someone to the hospital. Find out your family history and consider a gentle, preventive tonic like Pipsissewa.

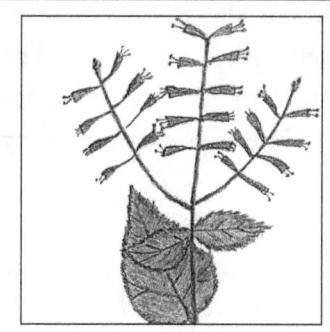

WOODS
Collinsonia canadensis

Stoneroot

Stoneroot is in the Mint Family, so it has a square stem. This plant is perennial and can grow up to four feet tall. It is fairly easy to recognize, as it has large, opposite, toothed leaves wider than they are long! The flowers are a greenish-yellow. The lower lip of the blossom is fringed and the stamins protrude (perhaps to entice wandering insect pollinators). The leaves have a lemony balsam fragrance, which also helps with identification.

You can use the fresh leaves as an external poultice for burns, cuts, bruises, or sprains. This would not be a good plant to chew in the field, as the fresh leaves seem to cause an upset stomach. This dilemma is no longer a problem after the leaves are dry. This is a large plant with large leaves, so it will be able to share its medicine without risk to itself.

An infusion of dry leaves, one teaspoon per cup of boiling water and steeped covered for ten minutes, is good medicine. You can sweeten the tea with honey and use it as a gargle for hoarseness or mild sore throat. The tea is also diuretic and is helpful for cystitis in the bladder or kidneys. The same tea also helps remove uric acid buildup and catarrh in the valves of the heart.

This is one of the plants helpful in preventing serious conditions. One of the chemical ingredients in Stoneroot is rosmarinic acid which is an anti-oxidant. Any plant that can help keep the valves of the heart from "congesting" is a good friend. If this condition occurs in your family, or if one of your elders is beginning to show symptoms, this might be a good tonic plant.

For stone prevention you could use Stoneroot leaves with Pipsissewa, and steep them together. If you want to use a root which needs to be prepared as a decoction (simmered), you could first simmer the root for the thirty minutes then remove the pan from the heat. Quickly add the leaves of the plant for a tea, then let the roots and plants steep, covered (off the heat) for the ten minutes needed to make your infusion. All that remains is to filter roots and plants through a cloth and the liquid is both a decoction and an infusion.

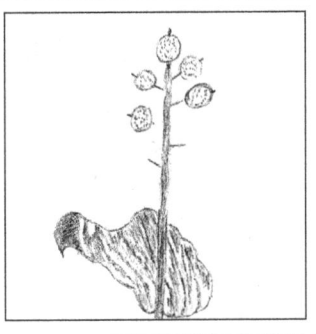

WOODS
Maianthemum canadense

Canada Mayflower

Canada Mayflower is a fascinating plant that grows very happily in the shade of the White Pines of the Northern Forests. It belongs to the Lily Family and the fragrance of the blossom lives up to this name. The plant itself is only about four inches tall, but it grows in colonies with many of its own kind. The plants are all interconnected by their shared root system.

The little Mayflower has two alternate, heart-shaped leaves along the stem. The blossom is a terminal spike of star shaped white flowers with four petals each. When the flowers are finished with their time of pollination, they form white berries with little spots. Over time the berries change to a pale red color. Its Indian name, "Agongosimin" translates as "Chipmunk Berry," and is very appropriate. The plant grows to the height where a passing chipmunk can sit on its haunches and take a nibble of the tart little berries.

The Canada Mayflower has a complex, perennial system of interwoven rhizomes. Some Canada Mayflower plants produce only one leaf, and these plants do not flower. These "helper" plants contribute their energy to the plants that do flower and contribute indirectly to the ongoing of their plant colony. The nutrients are actually shared through the root system.

This small plant has good medicinal sharing for people, too. A leaf infusion helps with headache and sore throat. This plant is a safe medicine choice for women who are pregnant. The Canada Mayflower leaves are diaphoretic and diuretic. This makes it a tonic for the bladder and kidneys.

In "congestive" conditions this plant helps remove excess mucus in the heart and throughout the vascular system. Not surprising it also helps with bronchitis, which is also a congestive condition. Canada Mayflower helps the body get rid of congestive waste wherever it occurs. This is a lot of medicinal activity from such a small plant. Canada Mayflower needs careful gathering so the leaf loss does not affect the strength and vigor of the colony. Usually the groups are big enough to help people and still have berries enough to take care of hungry little chipmunks. I really don't know if the little rodents are after the food value or if they need plant medicine for their own bodies.

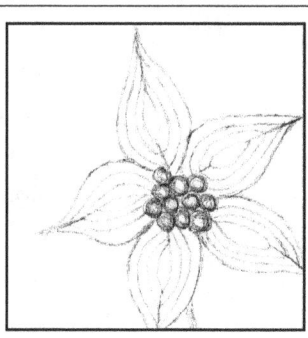

WOODS
Cornus canadensis

Bunchberry

Bunchberry is the smallest of the *Cornus* plants. The others are small trees, one of which is flexible enough to be the frame for a wigwam. This little Cornus plant loves the moist forest at the feet of the conifers.

Bunchberry grows from a cloning rhizome which allows colonies of this Cornus to burst into flower at the same time. The flower is white, with five good sized petals that surround a tight cluster of yellow-green flowers. The plants are insect pollinated, attracting bees and flies for help with this activity.

There are usually five or six oval leaves in a whorl around the flower. Sometimes though, if the plant is not going to bloom, it may only have four leaves in the whorl. Plants are very concerned with reproduction, so they waste no energy forming leaves for the fun of it. A flower needs the energy of sunlight, and is better fed by more leaves.

The Native People of the Great Lakes would gather the bright red berries, as they are abundant and dry easily for winter storage in their covered birchbark makuks. The berries could be cooked down into a kind of pudding or sauce to flavor stew, as well as provide vitamins during the winter months.

Medicinally the Bunchberry is also willing to share. The dried leaves provide a tea which helps with aches and pains, as well as difficulties with the kidneys or lungs. This is a tonic kind of medicine, gentle and effective.

It is good to find medicine in an abundant plant. There are many, Bunchberry plants growing among the Pines and Cedars. It is not a danger to the ongoing of the Bunchberry to gather leaves after the flowering time is ended. Bunchberry does not rival the Raspberries for sweetness, but the food energy is there in abundance for a hungry bird like the vireo, or chipmunks who like finding food near the ground where they can reach it.

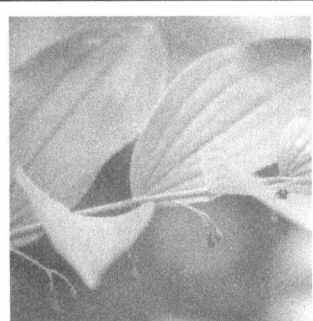

WOODS
Polygonatum biflorum

Solomon Seal

Solomon Seal is a perennial plant living alone or in small colonies. The arching stem supports long, slightly oval, alternate leaves. The veins are parallel like Plantain leaves. Greenish-white bell shaped flower pairs grow from the leaf axils under the stem. The flowers are well placed to allow easy access to the insect pollinators. Flowers and insects have a very intimate relationship that is good for both; food for the insect and pollination for the plant.

Solomon Seal grows about eighteen inches tall. The leaning stem allows the leaves to capture as much sunlight as possible in the wooded setting. The flowers transform to seed bearing, bluish-black berry pairs that drop later leaving empty stems to mark where they once grew on the plant. This is helpful for recognizing this plant later in the season.

The root is actually a thick, fleshy rhizome growing near the surface. When the plant was plentiful it was a food source for the Native People. It is this "root" that offers the medicinal gifting of Solomon Seal.

A root decoction can help with the pain of arthritis, rheumatism and gout. The plant is anti-inflammatory so it helps reduce the inflammation which is a part of these conditions. Swelling and pain are the noticeable factors, and it was a great gift to early herbalists to find a plant that could help with both conditions. These early herbalists also gathered carefully so that the Solomon's Seal would be there for the generations to come. They could not ask a plant for help with a healing and then bring about the extinction of the plant.

The root of this plant can also be used as a poultice for boils, wounds, serious bruises and broken bones that break through the skin. The resetting of broken bones was known to early healers, as well as the possibility of "bone fever." A warm poultice plus a cup of root decoction certainly helped with the pain and perhaps also helped with the healing of the bone. Solomon Seal and many other plants, are not considered "medically helpful" today. We are busily sending botanists to South America and ignoring the plants who still live where we live. Sigh.

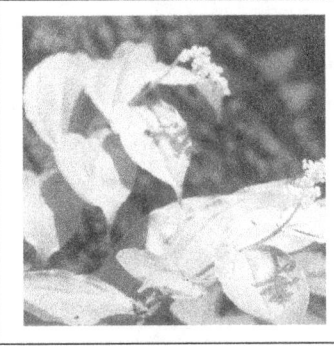

WOODS
Smilacina racemosa

False Solomon Seal

We are going to do the "botany thing" for this plant and call it by its Genus name—*Smilacina*. True this plant is similar in some ways to Solomon Seal, but it is not related in any way except appearance. This plant really deserves a name of its own.

Smilacina is perennial and grows to about twenty inches tall. The stem inclines so the leaves of this plant catch maximum sunlight, a good idea for a plant. The long leaves have parallel veins that alternate along the stem.

The stem itself is unique, as it zigzags a bit on the journey from flower to root. The flowering method is also unique and is the easiest method to tell which plant you are looking at. Smilacina has tiny white flowers that grow in a cluster at the top end of the stem. This full, fluffy cluster of flowers reminds me of Goldenrod.

The little berries that form from the blossoms are first white with brown speckles. Over time they turn a translucent red. Even after the fruit drops, or is eaten by a passing creature, the little flower stems are still there at the top of the plant.

The medicinal gift of this plant comes from the root. A mild root decoction (simmer for ten minutes) is good for lower backache, cramps, and headaches. It is diuretic and very helpful to the kidneys, especially during pregnancy when they must do extra filtering work. The root contains sitosterol which helps strengthen the heart and lower the heart rate.

These medicinal gifts are worth knowing. A plant that can be of help safely during pregnancy is a good thing. With Native American medicine the testing is not on laboratory rats who are given overdoses of isolated chemicals. The medicines were tested slowly and carefully by herbalists who only used them when given direction by Spirit. Over the years the herbalists would share the information so other people could also be helped. There was no payment for plant medicine, the healing was considered the Gift of the Plants. The herbalists would be given food gifts sometimes since their time was given over to working with plants for the People. This is why I do not sell herbs. I talk about plants so you can get them if you wish.

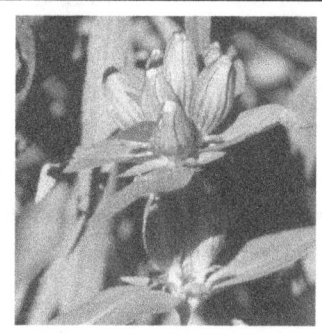

WOODS
Gentiana spp.

Gentian

Fringed **Gentian**, *Gentiana crinita*, is one of the first plants my herb mother sent me to find. "Go and see this plant, do not pick it, just look at it." It seemed a strange order but I went into the wet woodlands and when I found the plant I understood. It is very beautiful. A misty blue flower forms at the top of its own stem. It is shaped like a slender vase with four rounded purple-blue lobes that are deeply fringed. The blossom opens only in full sunlight and spreads its petals in four directions. There are lines of a deeper blue purple inside the flower. Gentian is an annual so it must reseed itself every year. I am grateful the flower is so beautiful, it is also appealing to bees and other winged pollinators.

Closed (or Bottle) Gentian, *Gentiana andrewsii*, also grows in wet woodlands, or along a shoreline where the trees give shade for part of the day. It is a perennial growing perhaps two feet tall. The blossom is a tightly closed deep violet blue flower with white stripes at the base. The color becomes deeper and more intense near the top of the flower. The flowers grow from the leaf-bases as well as at the top of the plant. It is a small cluster or, pair of flowers, that offer their beauty to passing humans and food to the bees. It sounds like I am fascinated by bees, but it is more serious than that. Our bees have been decimated by micro-organisms, and the number of native bees is dangerously low. We very much need the help of these "hummers" to share their honey and visit the flowers that offer them nectar in exchange for pollination.

Stiff Gentian, *Gentiana quinquefolia*, has tight clusters of blue tubular flowers growing at the top of a stout four edged stem. The leaves are oval and are attached directly to the upright stem of the plant. Each flower cluster has five blossoms displayed near the top of the plant stem.

There was a time when the root of this Gentian was used as a digestive tonic. It helped with food absorption especially in chronic wasting diseases. Since the Gentian are not an abundant plant, I would much rather find a more abundant plant to help with digestion and leave these flowers to their beauty and whatever purpose Gentian follow without my interference.

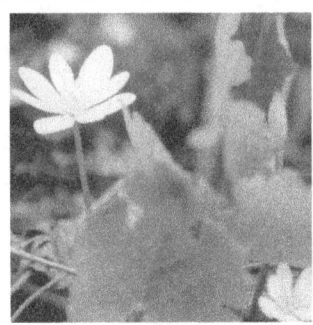

WOODS
Sanguinaria canadensis

Bloodroot

In the early days of Spring when it is the time of Trout Lilies, Spring Beauty, and Hepatica, it is also the time for **Bloodroot**. This is an unusual perennial. Bloodroot grows about ten inches tall and the flower begins almost before the leaves. The leaves look like deeply lobed White Oak leaves and are curled around the flower stalk, perhaps to protect it. A white flower with eight to twelve petals opens by day and closes up at night. The blossom has many gold stamins and is self pollinated. Perhaps the closing of the flower nightly helps with this.

The flower only lasts a few days, then the seeds form and are also protected by the curled leaves which grow tall enough to wrap around the seed case. The seeds are dispersed by ants who are willing to help the plant even in the chilly days of spring. Bloodroot is very specific about where it will grow, it forms colonies in the rich hardwood forests. Because we have lost so many of these forests, we have also endangered this plant. My herb mother asked me to be aware of this plant but not to gather it.

Sometime soon, I hope, when Bloodroot has found a way to increase in number, I would like to become better acquainted with this plant. Its Indian name, "Miskojiibik," means "Medicine Root," and it was very much a part of the healing ways of the People. The root itself has a red liquid which is almost the color of blood. When there were many forests, Bloodroot was a part of a cough syrup that was very helpful for asthma and bronchitis. My herb mother also used it with Curly Dock root for pernicious anemia.

There are health cautions about sanguinarine which is present in the root. It has been suggested this chemical is toxic and may cause glaucoma. If this is true, I have to wonder why this same chemical is used in commercial teeth whitening products.

Bloodroot belongs to the Poppy family. The seeds, if used as a medicinal, will cause a positive reading on a drug test. There is only a trace of the opiate compounds but I wanted you to be aware of this result. The chemical is also present in the root, perhaps a Mullein cough syrup would be less hazardous to your employment.

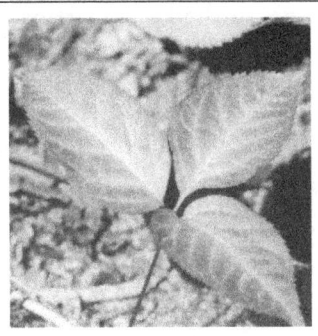

WOODS
Aralia nudicalis

Sarsaparilla

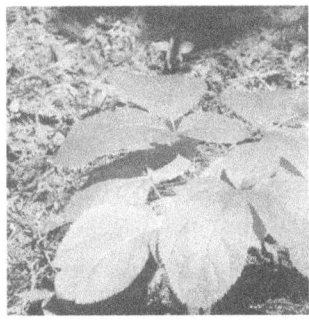

WOODS
Panax quinquefolium

Wild Ginseng

Wild Sarsaparilla, or *Aralia nudicalis*, is an interesting woodland perennial. The leaves are twice divided, and each grouping of three has three to five toothed oval shaped leaves. Where I have found the plant, the leaves have a coppery-brown shading mixed in with the green.

Like its Indian name, "Bebamabik," the "root runs horizontally under the ground." This root is fleshy and moist. The flower is an umbel (like an umbrella) on a long stalk, and stands clear above the plant. It is an easy access plant for flying insects to help with pollination.

The root has been used as a poultice for sores and burns, as it helps reduce swelling. The root also makes a nice tasting tea that can also help internally with stiffness and the pain of the conditions that require the poultice.

Wild Ginseng, *Panax quinquefolium*, is a Ginseng native to America. It is a perennial growing to two feet tall. Ginseng can live twenty to thirty years, but it is now rare from over harvesting. There are four to seven long somewhat oval leaflets. Like its cousin, Sarsaparilla, the leaves are toothed and the flower is an umbel of greenish-white flowers in a small round cluster. The seeds are red berries with two seeds.

At the top of the fleshy, white root is a rhizome, a runner that connects it to other Ginseng plants. Like other Ginsengs, this plant is medicinally active as a nervine and tonic to the body systems. It is also a nudge to the immune system. Ginsengs are restorative and raise the energy level of the body.

My herb mother taught that Ginseng is a man's medicine, that women would be better served by other plants. Siberian Ginseng is the only Ginseng I have used. The above ground parts of the plant are used, and it does not take the life of the plant. Please help the Wild Ginseng to restore itself and become plentiful in the woods.

Ginseng contains steroidal glycosides, sterols, and vitamin D. It is restorative but requires care in its use. Some people get headaches from taking Ginseng. If someone needs the help of Ginseng, try a small dose first and see if this plant is being accepted by the body. A tired body does not need more stress in the name of a cure.

If Ginseng is perhaps a plant for men, the next three plants are intended more for women. It is not discrimination, it is more that men do not have the parts which are the healing area of these plants.

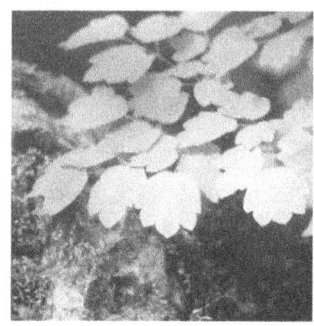

WOODS
Caulophyllum thalactroides

Blue Cohosh

Blue Cohosh is a perennial growing to about two feet tall. It is a distinctive woodland plant, its leaves and stem are covered with a bluish film. This is a lovely color and it is accented by the deep blue berries that form near the top of the plant. The leaves are compound mostly into threes: three leaflets with three lobes (usually).

Blue Cohosh blooms early before the leaves come out. The underground part is a root-rhizome. This is the part which is used medicinally, so it must be gathered with care for "the ongoing of the plant. Before any words about the healing aspects of Blue Cohosh are said, I write largely DO NOT USE DURING PREGNANCY.

It is the gift of Blue Cohosh to stimulate uterine contractions. This is a wonderful gift for a mother in childbirth who needs help with the process of birthing a child. The traditional medicine woman was aware of this plant and it was there in the birthing lodge to help with labor, and protect against inflammation of the uterus. This same gift also helps with excess menses and the cramping that can be part of the monthly cycle.

One cup of water and a teaspoon of dry Blue Cohosh root should be simmered for ten minutes, then filtered for drinking. For normal menstrual cramps I believe Crampbark (*Viburnum*) would be a better choice since it does not take the life of the plant.

There is research being done on Blue Cohosh. This plant contains steroidal saponins and alkaloids. It is estrogenic and it is also anti-inflammatory. Unfortunately it also seems to raise blood pressure (the problem with steroids).

For a woman who has already delivered her child this plant contains Potassium, Magnesium, Calcium, Iron, Silicon and Phosphorus. I was told it helps to alkalize the blood and urine (avoid uric acid - stone formation). Blue Cohosh is most specific with its help during the birth process. After delivery I would rather use Blueberries and Nettle tea to help the mother regain strength and energy.

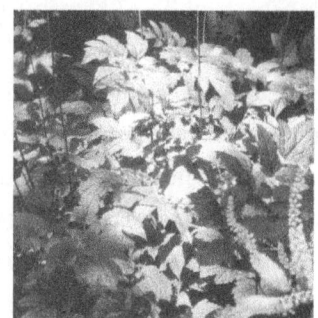

WOODS
Caulophyllum thalactroides

Black Cohosh

I do not know why this plant also has the common name "Cohosh," as it certainly causes confusion for people. The two plants have a different Genus and Species, and they don't look anything alike! Both do offer special help to women, but the nature of that help is also different. When searching for information about plants, or buying herbs from an herbal supplier, please request what is needed by the Latin Names so you will know you have the correct plant.

Black Cohosh is a very tall perennial. It grows three to eight feet tall! The leaves are sharply toothed and the end leaf has three lobes. The middle leaflet is always the largest. The white flowers grow on a long spike. Black Cohosh has a large, knotty root. A root tincture has been the best way to work with the gift of this plant. Some plants find it easier to release their medicinal qualities in alcohol. Scientists call it "alcohol soluble." This may be so, but there is also the fact this is not a yummy tasting root. With a tincture one can take the medicine by spoonful rather than by the cupful. Like Blue Cohosh, I will write DO NOT USE DURING PREGNANCY.

Black Cohosh is estrogenic, sedative, anti-spasmodic and anti-inflammatory. This plant can be helpful to a woman when she begins menopause. As you recall there are hormonal shifts in menopause not all that different from puberty—the body is not amused. Black Cohosh seems to help with hot flashes and other symptoms. These same gifts also help women who have difficult or painful periods. Black Cohosh has balancing gifts, it relieves pain, reduces inflammation and helps with sleeping difficulties.

Black Cohosh tincture is also anti-spasmodic and a mild cardiac stimulant, much safer than digitalis. If a person is having difficulty with rheumatism this plant may well be able to help with the swelling and with the pain factor.

Part of the teaching I am trying to share is how very specific the medicinal action of the plants can be. Black Cohosh may be anti-spasmodic, but the relief of cramping is mostly uterine. For a cough and the spasms of that condition, Mullein would be the better choice. There is no reason then to take the life of a Black Cohosh when Mullein will gladly share its leaves to help with bronchial spasms.

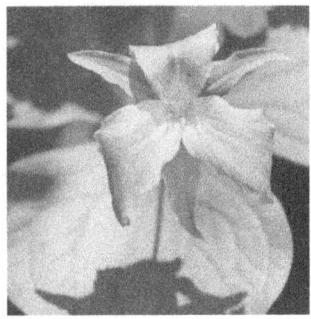

WOODS
Trillium erectum

Wakerobin

Red Trillium is a lovely perennial growing seven to fourteen inches tall. I know you have an image of me walking around in the woods with a yardstick measuring plant heights and marking them on a nearby tree trunk. I don't do this, I just try to give you the range I have seen.

This Trillium has showy red flowers that grow in threes. There are three sepals, three petals, and there are also three leaves if you want to take a look at the whole plant. The Trilliums have the help of bees and butterflies for their cycle of pollination. Somehow the plants which are part of the woman's cycle appear to have the phenomenon of *threeness* (the Celtic women say, "We knew that"). The fruit is a dark red, angular berry which later becomes a capsule. The seed capsules only germinate after lying dormant on the soil for two years. Before the flowers appear, the leaves are quite similar to Jack-in-the-Pulpit leaves. It matters which is which, so wait until the time of flowers to be certain. The medicinal gift comes from the thick, brown root. Once again I write...DO NOT USE DURING PREGNANCY. Strange that such woman specific plants would all have this warning, and yet it is the nature of the plant gift that makes this important.

Red Trillium contains steroids, steroidal saponins, steroidal glycoside, tannins and trillin. My herb mother used this plant medicine to induce labor. Sometimes a woman cannot get the birth process started even though the time has come. This Trillium also acts to cleanse the uterus after the birth. Its most important gifting, perhaps, is that it acts to stop internal bleeding. If there are problems after the birth a woman can easily bleed to death (unfortunately this still happens). To stop uterine bleeding the Trillium root is prepared as a decoction, with the addition of Cranesbill (Geranium Maculatum) root. Two teaspoons of each are simmered in one cup of water for ten minutes.

It is wise to see to childbirth in a hospital with the help of an obstetrician, or a midwife. However we do not know the way of the future. It is good these gifts of the Plants be known and remembered.

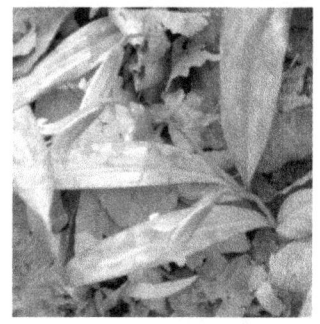

WOODS
Erythronium americanum

Trout Lily

Trout Lily has the Indian name "Numaebugoneen," which means "trout markings." The mottling on the leaves is similar to the speckles on the side of a trout. Trout Lily grows in large colonies with most plants reaching about a foot tall. This perennial plant often buds out from previous corms (tuberous root-like structures). There is a similarity of leaf pattern markings throughout the colony. Some of the Trout Lilies do not blossom but rather contribute their energy to the rest of the colony. Trout Lily blossoms in early Spring utilize the extra sunlight which reaches the forest floor before the trees leaf out. This plant is a sun lover, and the flowers turn throughout the day to follow the path of the sun.

The flower is yellow and grows on a long, nodding scape. It has six petals and is insect pollinated, or if that fails, self-pollinates. The Trout Lily is a survivor. It has its own little phosphorus cycle, as the roots draw phosphorus up from the soil, give it to the leaves, and then return the phosphorus to the Earth when the leaves fall to feed the next season of Trout Lilies. This little plant has strong relationship with the Sun and the Earth. It is not surprising it is both food and medicine for Bears.

Under the ground is a complex of corms. In early fall the bears dig the corms with their strong claws. Humans, usually in the form of an herbalist, gather leaves and corms. A leaf poultice is good medicine for slow healing sores. Both the leaves and the roots are anti-bacterial (for many kinds of harmful bacteria). A root tea, or infusion, is helpful for fever.

The corms are tasty for people, too. The bulbs can be boiled or fried. Bears eat them raw and have the full benefit of the medicinal gifting of Trout Lily as well as a tasty meal. Bears are the most like humans of all the woodland animals. They can stand upright for better vision and can harvest foodstuffs with their front paws. In a berry patch the bear just scrapes the berries off the plant and into his mouth. There are many stories of the Spiritual relationship that is possible with Bear. Bear is one of the original Clans of the People of the Great Lakes. Those who were Bear Clan were usually those who protected the village, or they were the herbalists who worked with medicinal plants. Bear is called "Mukwa," and you may see the word as the name of a boat, or a town, where people honor the strength and courage of Bears.

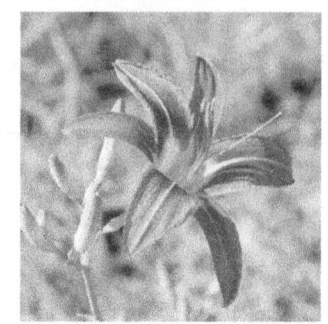

WOODS
Lilium philadelphicum

Wood Lily

Wood Lily, *Lilium philadelphicum,* grows tall and beautiful in the woodlands. It has deep reddish-orange flowers with black spots. Wood Lily can grow to three feet tall with lance shaped leaves growing in whorls along the tall stem.

Its Indian name, "Mashkodepin, meaning "Medicine Flower," tells about the awareness of the Indian People to what might be expected from this plant. Like the previous plants, this plant also can help with the birthing process. A tea made from the root helps to expel the placenta after the child is delivered. It is important this happen in a way that leaves no aftermath to cause infection. The same tea also helps with the fever which indicates trouble in the birth zone.

The Wood Lily flower was used as a poultice for spider bites. This also is helpful. You remember this same gifting comes from Plantain, in case the Wood Lilies are not in bloom.

The Michigan Lily, *Lilium michiganse,* also grows tall in the woodlands. The flower is a bright orange-red but the flower shape is very different from the Wood Lily. The flower itself is on a nodding stalk (it droops down) and the petals are "reflexive" (they curve back away from the stamins). The flower has small, freckle-size spots. The leaves are much like Wood Lily growing in whorls along a stem which can reach four feet tall.

A root tea made from Michigan Lily is helpful for stomach problems as well as dysentery. This tea helps the entire digestive tract. As we have talked about before, there is the connection between digestion problems and some forms of arthritis. Michigan Lily can help with some kinds of arthritis, and it is also willing to work with the aches and pains of rheumatism. This was a great gift for the People of the Great Lakes who lived their lives in the forests. Cold and dampness are hard on the muscles and joints, as any elder can tell you. Lilies enjoy the company of others of their kind. The woods wears large patches of these very lovely flowers.

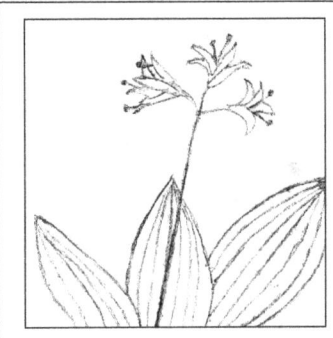

WOODS
Clintonia borealis

Bluebead Lily

This Lily is perennial and grows to twelve inches at its tallest. It has basal leaves (grow at base of stem) that are shiny and thick. **Bluebead** sends up a flower stalk with yellow-green flared blossoms. The fruit is a deep blue berry.

Bluebead is medicinal in its leaves and in its root. The fresh leaves make a good poultice for burns, cuts, and small infected areas of skin. They can also help an older cut that has trouble healing. The dried leaves make a tea which is a help for early diabetes before there is need for insulin, at the time when diet can help control the condition. For some people diabetes can be the result of being overweight, or it may set in as a person grows older. Many times a "borderline diabetic" can avoid the more serious problems that come with diabetes. Bluebead Lily, Bearberry, and other plants can be of real help with this, especially if we remember to ask them for the spiritual healing which can help the human spirit as well as the physical body.

The root also has medicine and is prepared as an infusion, (a tea). Most roots are used in a decoction, but the white starchy root of Bluebead does not require this. Like some of the previous plants, this Lily also offers to help with the birthing process. The root tea helps with labor and also helps prevent internal infection after the birth of the child. The root contains diosgenin which is anti-inflammatory and estrogenic. Bluebead root has been used in the research laboratories to produce hormones such as progesterone and testosterone.

I suppose this might worry some folks who do not realize humans have both these hormones. It is just that women have more estrogen and men have more testosterone. These hormones promote the well being of the reproductive processes. When a woman gets older the estrogen does NOT dry up, never to be heard from again. It is more that the body places this hormone, and other hormones, at a level suited to a body which is not producing children. Hormone levels are a part of the inner balance of the body, and we need them all through our lives. I believe an estrogen made from a plant is a better route than estrogen derived from the urine of a pregnant horse which is used in several prescription medicines. I also think the horse does not appreciate being kept pregnant to provide hormones for humans.

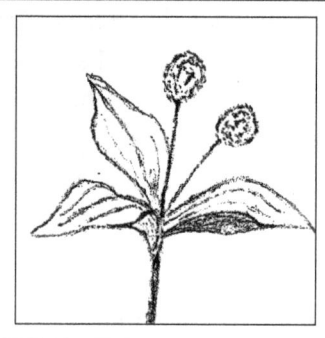

WOODS
Medeola virginiana

Indian Cucumber Root

This is the last of the woodland Lily Family I will talk about, though there are many more plants in the Lily Family. **Cucumber Root** is a perennial growing two to three feet tall. It is well named as it has a white tuber root which tastes very much like a cucumber. If there are a number of these plants in an area you may want to put down an offering and have a bite. It is better to wash and peel the root before tasting.

Cucumber Root has a tall stem with whorls of leaves, usually seven leaves to a whorl. The plants with only one whorl of leaves do not flower, the ones with two usually do have flowers. The extra leaves probably factor in the energy gathering system of the plant. Flowering has an energy cost to a plant, and the extra absorbed sunlight probably helps with this process. The oval leaves have parallel veins, very much like Plantain leaves.

The flower is a yellowish-green drooping blossom with red stamins. Cucumber Root is noticeable because the petals and sepals of the flower are reflexive (bending back and away from the stamins). After the flowering time a purple berry remains which holds the seeds for the future plants.

A tea or infusion made from the leaves and berries is good medicine for convulsions. It was used for small children who can go from feeling fine to having a very high fever in almost no time. Sometimes a high fever can trigger convulsions, because the child's system is not old enough or strong enough to deal with so much heat. Western medicine uses something like phenobarbital for this, but the Native Americans did not have this choice, so they asked the Plants for help. Indian Cucumber Root offered to help with this condition. It is a safe and gentle tea, and the People were very grateful for the medicine.

This is not so different from the gift of the Foxglove, whose digitalis gifting gave longer life to the Elders who had weak hearts. It is perhaps difficult for you to believe Plants can communicate their medicinal properties, and yet they do. It may be through a dream, a vision, or a ray of sunlight falling on a certain Plant. The Medicine Person who goes out to pray must be willing to hear the voice of the Plants. We have many medicines as gifts of the Plants and the herbalists who gather them.

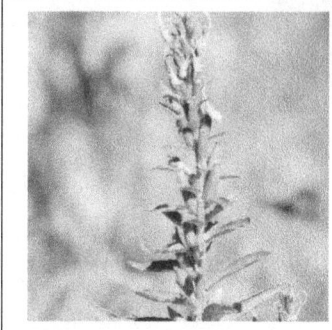

WOODS
Oenothera biennis

Evening Primrose

Evening Primrose is well named. *Biennis* is the species name and it is a biennial, like Mullein; a plant with a two year life cycle. The first year it produces many leaves, some along the stalk, some outward on branches. Most of the leaves form near the base of the plant. The nutrients drawn up by the roots are available for energy work in the leaves, and don't have to travel far. The second year the flowers come out at the leaf axils along the stalk and on the side branches.

The flowers are yellow with four wide petals and four drooping sepals. Why do they call it Evening Primrose? Because it blooms out after sunset! The pollinators for this plant are the evening insects. They have worked this out for the good of both insect and plant. It is good this plant continues blooming along the stalk over the summer season since the medicinal gift is in the seeds. What allows the ongoing of many flowers and plants are also of help to people.

Evening Primrose oil is astringent, nervine and sedative. It has been used for asthma and for whooping cough, as both have to do with spasms in the respiratory tract. We now have a vaccination for whooping cough, but we didn't when I was young enough to get it. Whooping cough is three months of trouble (strange sounding cough).

The oil also has gamma linoleic acid. There is much research being done with this. It seems to be a factor in hormone balancing in the body. It appears to help with metabolism disorders, PMS, migraine headache and arthritis. This sounds like a strange grouping of disorders but each condition is connected with tissues affected by the hormone system.

The balance of the inner systems of the body is just amazing. For instance, Migraines have a cyclic connection with a sudden change in hormone levels. For women this can be part of the menstrual cycle. For men it can be a by-product of an adrenaline overload. Either way hormones do not discriminate. Yes, metabolism also factors in, but it is guided by the hormone system. Metabolism is a strange word but the activity itself concerns how much energy we have available in our bodies. The body is a marvel, and it is a fine gift to have a plant that can help with this delicate balance.

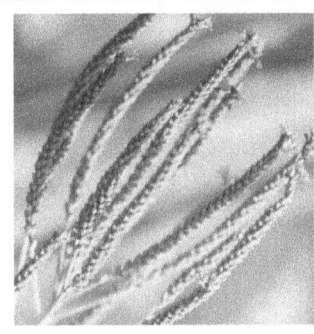

WOODS
Verbena hastata

Blue Vervain

Vervain is a squarish-stemmed perennial growing up to four feet tall, or a bit shorter depending on the soil conditions and the climate. I have found plants that are small in Wisconsin can be quite big in Ohio. I almost didn't recognize them! The common name, Vervain, appears to come from a Celtic phrase "Fer Faen" which translates as "drives away stones." I do not know if people from the British Isles visited America some time in the distant past leaving some of their words behind, but it wouldn't surprise me. Many people have been bothered by kidney and bladder stones and were very grateful to find a Plant which could help with this condition.

Vervain leaves are lance shaped and jagged toothed. They grow opposite each other on the stem and along the side branches. Sometimes the lower leaves of Vervain may have three lobes, which is perhaps a diversity the plant finds useful. The flowers are tiny blue-purple blossoms growing from the bottom to the top of the flower spikes. Sometimes the flower spikes are also branched producing even more little five petal flowers.

Vervain contains strong medicine in its leaves. I gather this while it is flowering, only picking a leaf here and there to allow the reproductive cycle of the plant enough energy to complete itself. Vervain tea (infusion) helps with diabetes especially when there is cloudy urine. The tea is a tonic protecting against stone formation. It also helps the liver rebuild when there is stress from poor waste disposal in the body.

Vervain tea seems to help with certain spasmodic ailments like a nagging cough, stomach cramps, dysentery, and even the intermittent fever that is sometimes a part of these conditions. It is possible that Vervain can also help with Epilepsy, but there are anti-seizure medicines now that make this unnecessary except in an emergency situation, such as being snowbound or lost in the forest. Some things still happen in spite of our civilized methodology. It is humbling that once in a while the weather does what it will and we can only wait until it is over. Vervain would be a good plant to keep in a glass jar, just in case.

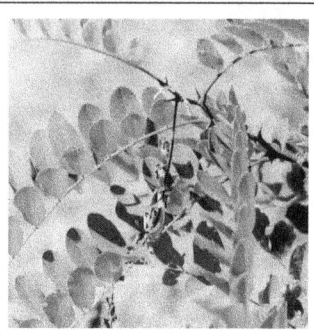

WOODS
Glycyrrhiza glabra

Licorice

Licorice is a perennial plant which is almost a shrub. It can grow up to five feet tall. Licorice has compound leaves with many pairs of dark green, smooth leaflets. The leaves are rather oblong and have tiny glandular dots. The bluish-purple flowers grow on fuzzy spikes. Licorice root is a dark, grayish brown color on the outside, and is usually wrinkled. The inside of the root is yellow and has a very sweet taste.

Gathering Licorice is interesting, as it is a bit like Ginseng. The best roots to gather come from plants over four years old. Not just any Licorice Plant will do, as the strongest medicine comes from the plants that do not bloom that season. The roots of the non-blooming Licorice plants retain more of their life energy and are able to share more of their healing gifts.

In general Licorice is anti-allergenic, anti-inflammatory, estrogenic, anti-bacterial and anti-convulsive. Licorice helps balance the body's metabolism, as it is a nudge to the adrenal glands which affect the entire endocrine system.

A root decoction (one tsp per cup of water, simmered for fifteen minutes) is a good way to prepare Licorice Root. A cup of Licorice Root can be taken three times a day for a short period of time, three to four weeks at most. Licorice is demulcent and can help with ulcers, bladder infections, harsh coughs and asthma. It is soothing to the lining of inflamed tissue. As a cough syrup, it is antitussive and the effects last longer than codeine.

However there are things you need to know about Licorice root. It may cause water retention in the body and thereby elevate blood pressure. No, you will not get a stroke from consuming Licorice, but care is needed for those with hypertension. Licorice allows for sodium retention and a loss of potassium. That is why it is only used short term, or not at all if the person already has high blood pressure. Those people need to remember our talk about Mullein and how effective that Plant can be for coughs and bronchitis. Many Plants overlap in their medicinal gifting. They all draw nutrients from the Earth and incorporate it into their living tissue. This makes for good choices for us, we who ask the Plants to share the medicine. I, too, have only begun to learn the ways of Plants.

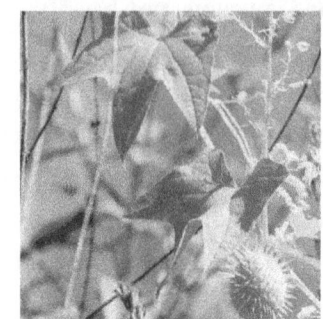

WOODS
Echinocyctis lobata

Wild Cucumber

Wild Cucumber is a climbing plant. It is found in fencerows, thickets, and sometimes up the walls of old farm buildings that have allowed wild plants to grow up around them. I have found the plant clinging by multiple tendrils to a small collapsed barn. Before I knew which plant it was, the prickly beauty of the seed pods asked to be photographed.

Wild Cucumber has maple-like leaves with five lobes. The leaf edges are toothed and the climbing tendency makes it clear this is not a tree. It has white flowers with six petals that grow in clusters from the leaf axils. The prickly seed pods look like little cucumbers. This is how it got the name Wild Cucumber. With that many prickles I did not try to sample it for taste. I had that experience with the fruit pod of a Prickly Pear Cactus. It may taste okay but removing the outer casing is painful.

The medicinal gifting of Wild Cucumber comes from the root. A root decoction is tonic for stomach problems. Wild Cucumber is a bitter, which is designed to help the digestive system. Bitters help the body put out juices which are needed to process our food. Sometimes with elders the body forgets to apply these digestive enzymes and the food can slip through the entire digestive tract without releasing its nutrients. It is also important to keep the food moving along the digestive pathway. Sometimes the system gets lazy and there is a "food traffic jam" which is not good. Then too much water can be removed, or things can ferment. Before we decided to put all our food in stores (so we would have to buy it back) these natural bitters were a part of our daily food intake. We seem to have forgotten all our plant food was "wild" at one time.

Wild Cucumber root decoction is also helpful for fever and chills. Some flu varieties go after the digestive tract and show no mercy. The Cucumber Root contains cucurbitacins which have shown promise as cytotoxic agents and may have anti-tumor activity. Since this plant medicine works in the stomach and intestines it might be a real help for those who have a family history which includes colon cancer. This kind of medicine is not prepared in a laboratory where chemicals are extracted until the medicine is no longer effective. It comes in the same balance that grows in the plant.

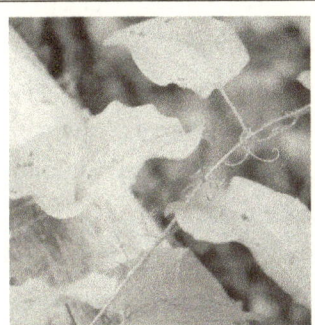

WOODS
Smilax rotundifolia

Cat Brier

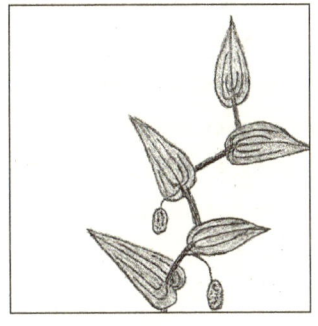

WOODS
Streptopus roseus

Twisted Stalk

There are six species of *Smilax* but **Cat Brier** has notable "cat claw" thorns (sharp and somewhat curved) along its stem. This woody perennial grows in thickets using tendrils to climb to its place in the sun. The leaves are rather oval and leathery. Cat Brier can hold its own against the other hardy thicket plants. After flowering it produces blue-black berries.

An infusion made with leaves and small stem pieces is very helpful for muscle cramps and symptoms of rheumatism. It is easy to harvest some leaves without damaging the life cycle of this plant. Whether it will be gentle with you in return may depend on placing an offering of Kinnik and asking for the medicine in a good way.

Cat Brier also may contain diosgenin which the pharmaceutical companies convert into steroidal compounds. In our bodies these hormones lower cholesterol, help alleviate the symptoms of stress and are anti-inflammatory. Since a simple infusion of leaves helps with rheumatism and muscle cramps, I have to suspect our bodies know how to work with the medicinal gifts of a plant without laboratory help (and cost!).

Twisted Stalk grows about two feet tall and the stem zig-zags in its growth pattern. The stem is hairy and the leaves attach right to the stem (no little stem of their own). The Indian name, "Agwingosbag," which means "ground squirrel leaf," reminds us of how the plant looks. With deep parallel veins, the leaf markings resemble the stripes on the back of a chipmunk. The little bell-shaped pink flowers become red berries along the twisted stem of the plant.

The leaves of the plant work like Yarrow in helping the body sweat out a cold or cough. In previous times, the root of this plant was steeped and the liquid became a compress for a sty, which is a red swollen eyelid caused by an infection.

Both Cat Brier and Twisted Stalk grow in the diversity of a natural woodland. It is hard for our society to leave the forest alone and allow the trees and plants to grow where they choose. We have control issues, you know. We move to the country and cut down or mow the very plants that make it a natural landscape…sigh.

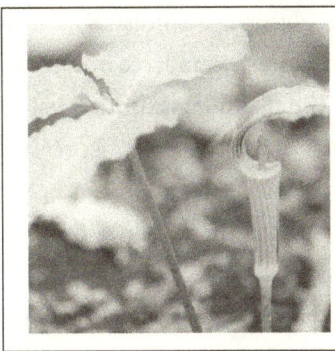

WOODS
Arisaema triphyllum

Jack-in-the-Pulpit

Jack-in-the-Pulpit grows in the moist places of a Maple forest. It is perennial and keeps company with Canada Mayflower and Sarsaparilla in the shaded places. This is a quiet woodland place with little wind to move the plants. The pollination is the work of insects, which for this plant is not easy. Sometimes the insect can get into the flower but can not get back out. The deep pitcher walls are slippery.

The plant grows about two feet tall and usually has two leaves with three leaflets each growing on long petioles. Since they are about the same height as the flower, this may provide a convenient resting place for flying insects. The flower is shaped like a slender vase and has a long overflap. The flower is solitary and is a greenish purple with beautiful stripes of deeper color near the opening. It is a pathway of color to guide the insects to the pollen.

Jack-in-the-Pulpit has the same kind of skill deer have. In a year of abundant food the deer will have two fawns. In a poorer year there will be only one fawn (or none). In a year of abundance the Jack-in-the-Pulpit, will produce two full leaves and a female flower. In a poorer year, it only produces one leaf and the flower is male. Yes, there is a higher energy cost in producing a female flower. If it is an impossible year, then the corm (root) waits for the next year. Jack-in-the-Pulpit has the ability to have a male flower one year and a female flower another year. It amazes me that a plant can be so flexible with its annual identity.

Most of the plant parts of Jack-in-the-Pulpit are toxic. It contains oxalate crystal which should not be taken internally. Even the root can cause a rash and it needs to be dried before using the corm to make a poultice. This poultice (use glycerin to moisten) has a healing effect on boils and on ringworm. Those who have boils may want to get acquainted (carefully) with the healing gift of this plant. Those who do not have these difficulties can benefit from just seeing the beauty of this unusual plant.

After the growing season the plant foliage dies back and what remains is a stem with an egg shaped cluster of red berries. That part of the plant does not resemble the flower in any way. It is good to know the way of plants at all times of the year.

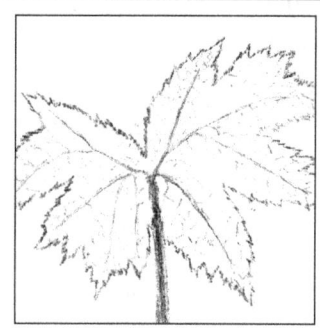

WOODS
Hydrastis canadensis

Golden Seal

Golden Seal in the wild has become rare, even endangered, from over harvesting. I buy this root from an herbal supply company that plants and harvests the root, so the plant will continue. It is expensive, and it ought to be. It is the place of last resort for certain conditions. Sometimes a profit oriented herb store will advertise Goldenseal for every little thing, since it is expensive and this brings in more money. Whatever the situation needs herbally, this plant should be the last choice. My herb mother told me it was unwise to begin with the strongest plant. As with certain antibiotics today, overuse has led to the development of drug resistant bacteria. I would not want to see that happen for this plant.

Goldenseal is a perennial plant usually about ten inches tall. It has a single hairy stem and produces two alternate leaves. The leaves are compound with five leaflets each. The leaflets are oval, deeply toothed and are a deep green color. The flower is a pinkish white solitary with three sepals and many green stamins. The fruit is a red berry similar to a raspberry. The root is a yellow-orange rhizome. Most often I use the powdered root in a gelatin capsule.

Golden Seal root is antibiotic. It contains hydrastin and canadine which reinforce the immune system. Do NOT take Golden Seal during pregnancy. The root medicine is anticatahhal, hepatic, and anti-bilious. It helps the mucus linings throughout the body. I have used this root in combination with powdered Myrrh gum to help with tuberculosis. The woman had AIDS and her immune system was having difficulty with infections that ordinarily do not affect the body. I would also use Golden Seal for serious problems in the kidneys and liver.

Please do not think I would do away with Western Medicine, as it is very effective in many conditions. I only offer help where nothing else has improved a person. Usually these are the chronic, or ultimately hopeless conditions that happen to some people. This is why I talk on and on about prevention. The best cure is not to get a sickness at all. This is where plants do their finest work. Tonic plants, not Goldenseal, are willing to help with many illnesses if your family history indicates a tendency.

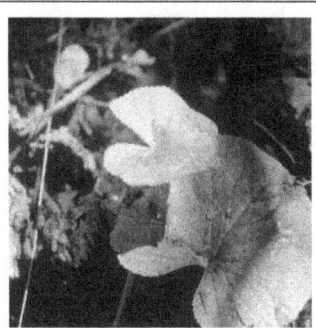

WOODS
Asarum canadense

Wild Ginger

Here is a plant whose Indian name, "Namepin," which means "Sturgeon Potato," refers to the great prehistoric fish who is known to the People as "The Spirit of the Great Lakes." This Spirit is not an individual fish, but the Spirit or Essence of Sturgeon. This Spiritual concept is a part of the Philosophy my herb mother believed. She would say, "All things are natural, the spiritual and the physical are always present in all things that exist." The Spirit of Sturgeon is a part of the Medicinal Gift of this Plant.

Wild Ginger is very similar to its domestic cousin, though I think it has more *character*. At the base of a hardwood tree you'll find a plant with velvety leaves. They are deep green. Plants growing in the shade seem to have a darker green color, since the plant makes more chlorophyll to absorb as much sunlight as possible. The leaves have a heart shaped base. The leaves are hairy on both sides and the stem is hairy. It is a furry little plant. The root is a rhizome joining many clumps of plants. It is easy to gather some of this root without damaging the "village" of Ginger. There is no doubt this is the right plant, as it smells like Ginger!

The root is antibiotic, and is a good internal friend. It contains aristolochic acid which has anti-tumor capacity. You know you are living right when the food you eat is also a medicine that can give good health. There was a time when many of the plants we are talking about were staples in the diet of the People. We have since hybridized our food into tidy little commodities that look good in styrofoam containers. I'm not sure we have done such a clever thing. In reality our vegetables grow in the ground. The problem is we think anything that grows in the soil is dirty. Getting dirty is dreaded as the "ick factor" which we caution our children against, but which doesn't help.

For motion sickness I like to combine powdered Ginger root with a little Cinnamon. It goes easily into gelatin capsules and works very effectively. The capsules are easier to explain to other travellers than chewing on a piece of root. I used to think I didn't get seasick until I travelled on a big ferry boat. I can do the up and down part, its the side to side roll that makes me uncomfortable. Thank you, Wild Ginger.

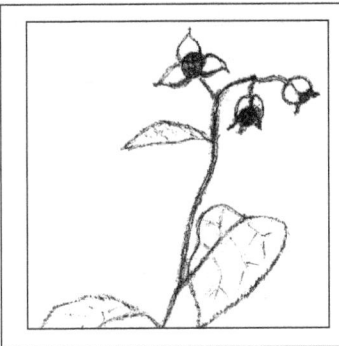

WOODS
Celastrus scandens

Bittersweet

Bittersweet can grow up to fifty feet tall, which is very tall for a woody climbing vine with no tendrils. The Indian name for this plant is "Bimakwad," which means "twisting around." It has slender, flexible green twigs that let the plant climb up until it reaches sunlight. The leaves are alternate, light green, finely toothed ovals with pointy tips.

It is easiest to identify after it has produced a fruit capsule. The outer covering is orange but splits to show the red seed cover underneath. This plant is now protected from harvest, but there was a time when it was a common fall decoration. I am grateful Bittersweet is protected, and I am also pleased it shares its autumn beauty with all who walk by, and remains alive to do this year after year.

Bittersweet will utilize insect pollinators, or it can contentedly clone itself if needed. Parts of this plant are toxic, especially the berries. I was told the Native Americans used the inner bark of this plant as a winter survival food by pounding dry outer bark to powder, then cooking it into a soup. I hope there will always be other foods to keep us alive during the winter.

There is a Nanabooshoo story about the origins of this plant. One cold winter day Nanabooshoo, son of the West Wind, and an Anishinabe woman, was walking across the ice. He heard something rattling behind him and turned to see what was making the noise. As could only happen to Nanabooshoo his intestines were dragging on the ground, they were partially frozen and making noise. Nanabooshoo broke off the frozen parts and threw them over a tree. "This shall be for the good of future relatives," he said, and it became Bittersweet.

My herb mother said the root bark in a decoction was diuretic and brought on sweat. Since Yarrow also does this, it seems the safer choice. However, I listened again when she said the raw bark was also a good poultice for skin cancers. It is not toxic to the birds who eat the seeds and then plant Bittersweet in other places with their droppings. I do not think I will be able to research this plant since it is protected. However, its beauty is there in September to remind us to prepare for the snows of Winter.

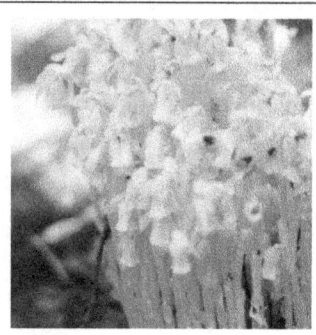

WOODS
Monotropa uniflora

Indian Pipe

Indian Pipe is a fascinating woodland plant. Just when things begin to make sense along comes the little colony of ghost plants. They are a translucent white. What once were leaves are now white scale-like leaves along the stem. This plant gave up chlorophyll to go at things in its own way. This is a perennial saprophyte.

The roots of this plant mesh with the below ground mycorrhizal fungi that connect with the roots of nearby green plants. I suppose this is opportunistic of the little plant, but it is effective. Indian Pipe grows in the moist, deeply shaded areas of the forest. The white flowers droop until they are pollinated (probably by a wandering insect) then the flower stands straight up even after the plant turns black. Indian Pipe follows the usual life process of a fungus. I have found this plant in Pine forests and also in the mixed woodlands further south.

It is the purpose of this plant, as with the other true fungi, to recycle the fallen organic matter of the forest. All the important minerals which are trapped in fallen logs and plant parts, as well as animals who have left this cycle, are reduced to their original state and are then available for the next generation of growing things. Without this help the future beings would starve. This is one of the dilemmas caused by clear cutting a forest. Almost all organic matter is held in the trees and plants. If this is not returned to the soil nothing will grow in the place! I salute the hard working fungi.

Indian Pipe is quite rare now because of changes in the forest lands. When the plant was abundant this plant shared its medicinal gift with us. A tea made from the "roots" is nervine and sedative as well as antispasmodic. It was one of the plants used for those prone to convulsions, or epilepsy. My grandmother mentioned the plant helped to sharpen vision. If the plant begins to thrive sometime soon I would wonder if it might be helpful for cataracts. Spirit willing this may one day be tested.

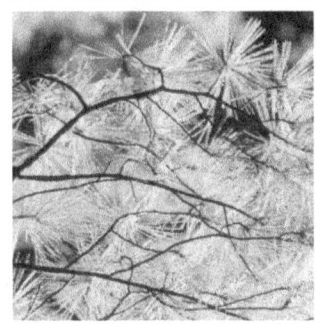

WOODS
Pinus strobus

White Pine

White Pine is a magnificent tree, and can live up to three hundred years. It prefers a sandy loam soil but can easily adapt to dry sand or swamp. The White Pine is slow-growing at first, as the young pines enjoy the shade of taller trees in the beginning. When it has grown a bit, it can then accelerate and grow as much as two feet a year.

Young White Pines have smooth, greenish brown bark, and the elders have gray bark with deep furrows. The branches grow out from the trunk in whorls of five. The spacing between the whorls can tell you what kind of year the tree has had. Most noticeable are the clusters of soft, blue-green needles that dance in the wind. White Pine has a deep relationship with the wind. There is a song as the breeze moves through the needles, and the tree depends on the wind for pollination.

The pollen and seed cones are on the same tree, they grow in the upper branches where the wind can reach them easily. The cones need two years to mature. It is only after that much time that the cones are released by the action of the spring winds. The White Pine often shares space with the Eastern Hemlock and the mixed hardwoods at the edge of the boreal forests. White Pine cones can also be germinated by fire (like the Jack Pine). In the eighteen hundreds there were many White Pine. It was the first tree to be lumbered off since the logs would float on the river that would then carry them to market.

The White Pine is very generous with its animal neighbors. It provides good nesting places for hawks and owls with branch spacing that allows room for large wings. The cone seeds are food for many birds and squirrels. A squirrel can strip a cone in less than a minute! Squirrel also helps the Pine by burying cones.

Humans have also been gifted. The inner bark can be pounded into flour for winter food. The pitch makes an excellent inhalant for coughs, when placed on heated rocks. It can also be used as a warm compress for sore muscles or rheumatism. The pitch is also a waterproofing sealant for canoes, wigwams, and storage makuks. White pine will continue to exude sap for a year after it is cut. I have gathered pitch where there has been lumbering, scraping pitch into an old glass jar. Rubbing alcohol cleans the knife.

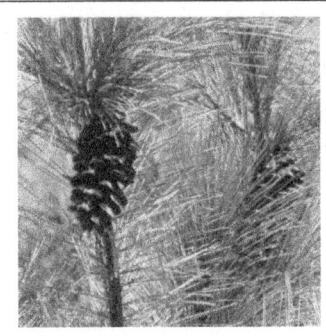

WOODS
Pinus resinosa

Red Pine

Red Pine has the common name "Norway Pine," though it does not come from Norway. Rather it is indigenous to North America, named for the town of Norway, Maine, where an early settler saw the Red Pines and was reminded of the trees in Norway. Red Pine shares space with Jack Pine, Aspen, and Oak trees. It has thick bark and is fire germinated where it can fill the burn area with its children.

Red Pine likes sandy, gravelly soil so it is comfortable in the glacial till of the northern Great Lakes area. The trees are tall and straight, growing up to two feet a year, some reach a hundred feet tall! Red Pine is self pruning; the lower branches drop off leaving the upper branches and needles in the sunlight. The needles are four to six inches long growing in pairs. These needles do not bend, rather they "snap" when bent. This may help you identify the Red Pine. The needles last up to three years before they drop and are replaced. The cones are oval with their scales spaced so the wind can move between them for pollination.

I find it fascinating that trees, which we think of as non-intelligent, have worked out such wonderful ways to live in their area of choice. Red Pine is evergreen so it has produced sheathed, weather resistant needles that last for years. The roots spread easily through the stony soil. It can reproduce by wind or by fire. Fire is a common phenomenon where the ground is covered with resin coated needles and branches. The thick, flaky, red-brown bark protects the tree from fire. The needles safely grow on the upper branches, and fallen cones germinate by the fire that melts off their coating of pitch. Red Pine is a tree perfectly designed for where it is and what it does. Amazing that this should be an evolutionary accident.

I have worked with Pine pitch, as it makes a great inhalant for colds and coughs. It will incorporate with oil and beeswax to make a vapor rub. I melt the pitch in an old glass jar warmed in a kettle of gently heated water. The old pitch jar is then empty for future gathering. I keep one in the car for the finding of more Pine pitch. The Pine pitch salve is also antiseptic and makes a good wound dressing for cuts or burns. Red Pine sawdust is also very aromatic, and makes a fine dream pillow. A dream pillow is a nice use for scrap pieces of flannel, it is very fragrant.

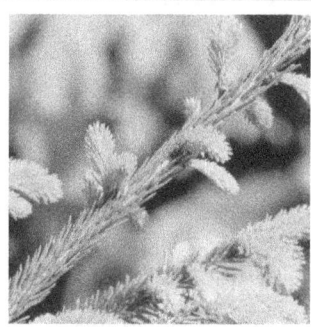

WOODS
Picea glauca

White Spruce

White Spruce is adaptable. It keeps company with Balsam Fir, Red Maples, Birches, Aspens, and Pines. Together these trees make a nice looking, balanced northern woodland. White Spruce tolerates sun or shade, wet or dry soil…it just grows, up to eighteen inches a year! During its life cycle White Spruce can reach seventy feet tall, and like the Red Pine, it prunes itself, dropping the lower branches. The bark is an ash gray color with scaly plates. It is bark with character, but is not designed to deal with fire.

The stiff, pointy little needles are singly attached (not in pairs, or groups). The needles wind around the twigs filling them nicely. The overall growth pattern and branch spacing makes the Spruce a fine looking evergreen tree. How will you know the White Spruce from the others? If you bruise some needles it has a nasty smell, it has a nickname "skunk spruce."

The birds and animals are not bothered by the needle smell. In winter food is hard to come by and Spruce is a welcome provider. The birds also seek out the White Spruce as a well protected nesting site. Woodpeckers, chickadees, and finches raise their babies in the Spruce branches. The number of bird residents goes up when there is an outbreak of insect pests. White Spruce lets these nesters clear the insects from its branches. It is a nice balance which the forest figured out with no help of the DNR.

The cones form over the summer and drop in the fall. The Spruce has worked out a clever strategy to fool the seed eaters who might eat all the seeds from the cones. It only produces cones with many seeds about every four to six years. With this pattern the seed consumers go elsewhere to do most of their eating.

The Native People used a smudge of fresh needles as a fumigant when there was a disease that might contaminate their wigwam. They may not have had a word for bacteria but they knew that the "unseen ones" were a cause of sickness. Otherwise their relationship with Spruce was for the making of canoes. The long slender roots made strong lacing for the sides of the canoe, the pitch of the Spruce made an excellent patching glue.

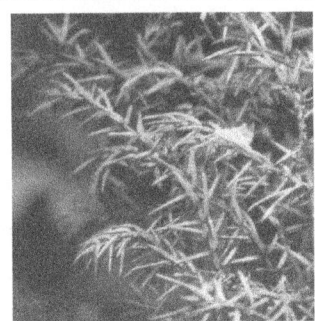

WOODS
Tsuga canadensis

Hemlock

This is not "poison Hemlock," but an evergreen that loves the moist areas of the woods. **Hemlock** casts a blue shadow, the boughs filter the light of the entire spectrum, except blue. This same filtering phenomenon makes the deep water of lakes appear blue.

Hemlock can live up to six hundred years, although two hundred is more common. It grows to about seventy feet tall and has a ragged crown. Hemlock boughs are flat and the needles are similar to Balsam Fir but Hemlock needles have little stems. The needles are about half an inch long and are yellowish-green on top with two white lines underneath. Once my grandmother watched a deer hunter steal a Hemlock tree from the woods for a Christmas tree. She knew the crime would not go unpunished. Hemlocks have very fragile needles, so she knew the tree would be almost bald by the time he got it home!

Hemlock has widespread, shallow roots. It is vulnerable to fire and drought. Perhaps this is why it chooses to grow in the wet areas of the woods. The parent tree absorbs so much of the ground moisture that the cones germinate better if they fall away from their mother. Since the cones drop in winter there are many hungry squirrels who will take care of dispersing the seeds.

The Hemlock twigs are very flexible and turn away from the wind. The flat boughs catch and hold snow so a Hemlock forest is a good place for deer to winter over. Some winters the snow is so deep it is hard for the deer to find food, so they eat the Hemlock boughs. Porcupine also loves to dine on Hemlock, although he goes up the tree to nibble the upper twigs.

The People of the Great Lakes used Hemlock needles for a winter tea, and used the dry inner bark pounded into a flour to thicken soup. The cooking makuks were always near the fire and the stew varied with what was available on a given day. Hemlock was both seasoning and medicinal as it kills *E. Coli bacteria*. When food is medicine the People stay healthy. Fresh inner bark is styptic, meaning it will stop bleeding. A needle and twig tea offers Vitamin C and a good medicine for diarrhea. The deep cold of winter was a time for both human and animal, to turn to the evergreens for food and medicine to stay alive.

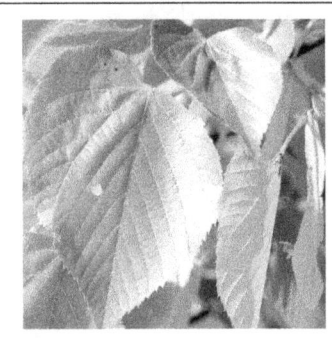

WOODS
Tilia americana

Basswood

Basswood flowers make delicious honey! The tree flowers in April before the leaves appear. The bees welcome the early blossoms and the tree "hums" with bees. It is good for the bees and very good for the ongoing of the Basswood tree.

Basswood has wide, heart-shaped leaves. The leaves are not even at the base, one lobe is usually longer than the other. The top of the leaf is dark green, and the underside lighter green but shiny like the top side. Along the midrib under the leaf there are fuzzy red hairs. This must protect the leaf in some way, but I don't know for sure. In fall the leaves turn a mottled yellow. It is nice contrast with its forest mates, the Maples and Ash trees.

This tree likes company, so it usually grows in clumps of four or five trees. The straight trunks grow quickly reaching to seventy feet tall. The seeds are round, and look like fuzzy peas. The seeds stay on the tree all winter providing welcome food for squirrels and quail. These sturdy little seeds stay viable up to three years waiting to bring on another generation of Basswood trees.

The Native People of the Great Lakes used the inner bark fibers to make strong lashing for canoes and wigwams. These People wandered through the seasons so a wigwam home that was easy to build was very helpful. They used young Cornus trees tied with Basswood fibers and an outer covering of Birchbark.

The wood of the Basswood is soft, great for carving (I have small hands, hardwood is too much for me). Sometimes a large section of tree will fall with the inside already hollow. A section of Basswood with leather covering the ends makes a drum with an interesting sound.

Basswood is closely related to the European Linden that produces lime blossoms for a relaxing tea. Basswood, which is also called the American Linden, may also make a nice tea. I have never asked the bees to move aside so I could find out. I have tasted Basswood honey and it is delicious. The tree draws up calcium, potassium, magnesium, and phosphorus from the ground. When the growing season ends in late fall these minerals are returned to the Earth with the falling of the leaves. This litter decomposes to become food for the next cycle of growth, food for the trees and for other plants.

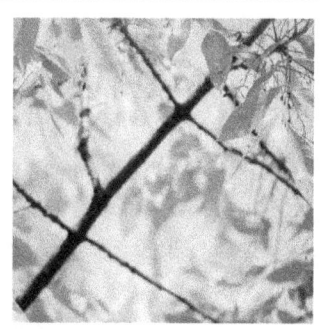

WOODS
Fraxinus americana

White Ash

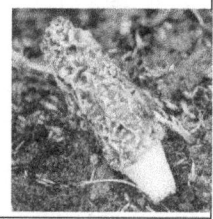

Ash is a tall tree with opposite branches. The opposite branches are most noticeable in winter when the bare branches are profiled against the sky. Ash twigs and buds are stout and covered with thick bark, well dressed to endure the cold and the winds of winter. The leaves are compound with seven finely toothed leaflets.

Ash is a "wind tree." It is pollinated by wind. Also the light, canoe paddle shaped seeds are distributed by the summer winds. Ash trees enjoy their own company and grow in groups. The male and female flowers grow on separate trees. I believe there is an energy saving by only producing the flowers of one sex, rather than both. The Ash grows quickly up to eighty feet tall. The trunks are straight with light gray colored bark. Ash grows deep roots and the stump will sprout again even after cutting.

The deep red leaves fall early in Autumn. Remember the story about leaf color—red leaves mean high levels of sugar in the leaves. With the deep root system there is also nitrogen in the fallen leaves. The soil around an Ash tree becomes very rich, so an old Ash forest is a good place to look for "Morels," those wonderful delicious mushrooms. Morels are the reason butter was created…totally delicious cholesterol!

The Native People used Ash for many things. As the Ojibwa name, "Aagimaak" suggests, Ash makes good snowshoe wood. The young overcrowded saplings were harvested after an offering of Kinnik, and carefully trimmed and bent into snowshoes. I have made snowshoes, and I urge you to bend the Ash stems very slowly! I soaked the branches in the bathtub, as warm water helps with flexibility (it works). Snowshoes made it possible for the hunters to go out into the deep snow forests and hunt food for their family. During the winter the People spread apart in the forests so the animal populations would be able to support the hungry people. Ash also made good sled runners to carry the deer home. In summer larger branches were carved into canoe paddles that were light weight, but strong. The women pounded Ash logs to remove the outer bark. The inner bark peeled off in splints which they could weave into baskets. A family needed baskets to store dry clothing and other sundries.

WOODS
Quercus alba

White Oak

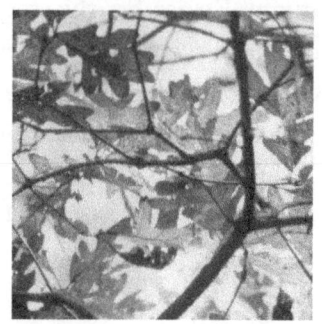

White Oak likes hilly, upland country. It grows happily with Hickory, Ash, and Walnut, or further North with the Aspen, Maples, and Pine. White Oak grows slowly. It sinks a deep taproot and can live over five hundred years! White Oak has wide branches and a short, stout trunk. With a killing frost the leaves turn a deep purple-red color.

The leaves have rounded lobes and hang in clusters at the end of the twigs. The rounded lobing on the White Oak varies from wide lobes to narrow lobes, to almost no lobing at all. The leaves are dark and shiny green on top fading to pale green underneath. The acorns mature in one growing season. The acorns are sweet. They are just short of an inch long and often hang on the tree in pairs. The acorn meat is high in protein, carbohydrates, and fat, and is the preferred acorn of squirrels and people.

The Native Americans of the Great Lakes called this tree "Mitigomin" which means "tree with good acorns." The People did not grow wheat or oats to use as flour for bread. Rather they utilized what was gifted to them by the White Oak, acorns that could easily be ground for making nutritious bread. White Oak acorns do not need to be leached, as the tannin level is much lower than the Black Oaks. This kind of bread may sound strange and yet we pay extra for nut bread in the store.

The White Oak does not produce acorns until it is about fifty years old. There is an abundant crop every four to ten years. This staggering of abundance has developed to protect the tree from insect pests who would otherwise get used to a yearly diet of acorns.

It is not only humans who prefer the white acorns. They are also food for bears, raccoons, deer, and white-footed mice. The acorns left behind by these eager consumers germinate quickly...wise tree.

Oak wilt is a condition which is dangerous to this tree. It is transmitted from tree to tree where their roots come in contact underground. In some yards all the oaks may be lost. In a diversified forest the oaks are far apart and do much better.

The inner bark has been used in an infusion for diarrhea, excess mucus and for bleeding. There is enough tannin in the bark to make the infusion styptic and antibacterial. There is more research needed on the antiviral and antitumor properties of this inner bark.

Since many animals choose to eat the acorns of the White Oak, there would not be enough acorns to feed the People through a long, hungry Winter. They turned to the Oak to gather the necessary acorns.

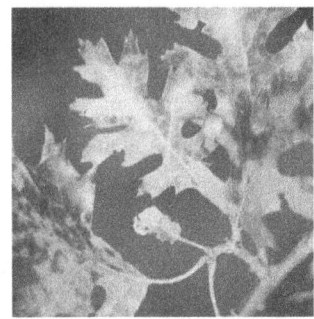

WOODS
Quercus rubra

Red Oak

Red Oak belongs to the Black Oak group. It has deep lateral roots, and lives to three hundred years, it is born to grow! It will resprout from cut stumps, and the high tannin content of the leaves and bark keep it safe from most insect predators (except the walking stick). Red Oak even produces phenols in its leaves to fight off the gypsy moths. This discourages the moths, with help from nuthatches, vireos, redstarts, and orioles who eat their share of the pests.

The Red Oak is food and shelter for many birds; including crows, turkeys, woodpeckers, blue jays, pheasant, and grouse. These are birds that stay North through the winter. The grackles must believe in the ongoing of the Oaks, as they have developed a palate keel inside their beaks just to open the acorns.

The Native Americans called this tree "Wisugimitigomic," which means "Bitter Oak." The acorns of the Red Oak required one of two solutions for leaching out the excess tannin. Sometimes the acorns were cooked by bringing water to a boil and changing the cooking water four times. Or, if the harvest was plentiful, they put the raw acorns into woven cedar bags and let these acorns soak for a year in the clear water of a spring. There is a spring in Upper Peninsula Michigan called Kitchitikippi which maps call Big Spring. My herb mother went to this place to get water for the making of certain medicines. While she explored the area she found several old woven bags of acorns which had been left there to soak. Gathering acorns and soaking them is much less work than gathering enough fire wood to boil the acorns four times.

The Red Oak also has a layer of inner bark which is anti-bacterial and will stop bleeding (styptic). This offers a good band-aid for cuts or scrapes.

Red Oak is a favored nesting place for squirrels. It is also known to give shelter to black bears. The Red Oak only grows to about sixty feet this far North, but it is a strong enduring tree that continues to hold its place in the mixed hardwood forests. The Red Oaks hybridize easily so the leaf lobes vary, but look for the familiar pointed leaf tips.

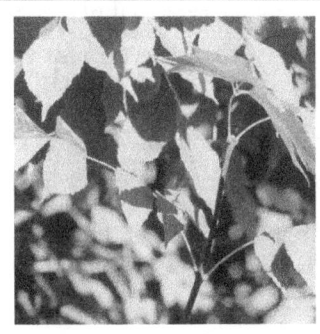

WOODS
Fagus grandifolia

Beech

There is a Biome, or region, called Maple-Beech Complex. These two trees have worked out their relationship. First one tree will take over the canopy of the forest. After a time the other will grow up to replace it in a fairly smooth cycle of dominance, each taking a turn at filling the high place.

The slow growing **Beech** is shade tolerant and keeps company with the Sugar Maples waiting for its time in the sun. Beech grows to eighty feet tall and can live up to four hundred years. Beech leaves are shiny green, pointed and have very straight veins. The bark is smooth and steel gray in color. This tree is very thin skinned and is vulnerable to fire or deep frost. But this is also a persistent tree. The shallow side roots sprout into colonies of young trees while the deep taproot continues feeding the parent tree.

The Beechnuts are marvellous food and the animals know this as well as people. The blue jays, squirrels and chipmunks scramble through the Beech trees dropping nuts to the forest floor. Grouse and turkeys are happy to harvest any nuts they can locate on the ground. In fall, there may well be claw marks from a black bear who thinks the oil rich nuts are just right for a before winter snack. Even wood ducks and porcupines share in the feast. Porcupine will den in the Beech tree and have nuts to eat through the winter.

For the People, Beech nuts were a winter staple also. After roasting, the spiny bract was removed. The whole nuts could be cooked with corn soup, or they could be crushed and boiled to release the oil. The oil floated and was skimmed off and saved. The remaining Beech nuts were then dried and ground into an energy rich flour.

Dry roasted nuts would store for winter in a covered makuk providing food all through the Winter. The time of fall harvest was very important, especially when the trees provided good rich nuts.

As an infusion, the bark is good for lung infections. During the growing season a leaf decoction is a good sterile treatment for burns or cuts. The medicine of choice for such conditions was the one that was available at the time of injury. Balsam Fir sap was stored for burns that happened over the winter. The plants provide what is truly needed for life.

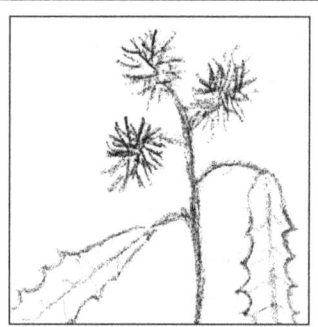

WOODS
Castanea dentata

American Chestnut

South of the sand line in the states around the Great Lakes there are still a few isolated stands of **Chestnut** trees. This tree can reach eighty feet tall, rubbing shoulders with Oaks and Hickories. The leaves are big; six to eight inches long. The yellow-green leaves droop on their stems and they are coarse toothed. The veins are parallel and a vein ends in each tooth of the leaf.

In mid-summer the Chestnut produces flowers, with staminate flowers (male) on one stalk and pistillate (female) flowers on a nearby stalk. The wind moves through the leaves and helps with the pollination. The resulting fruit is a spiny bur that covers two or three edible nuts. They are good raw or roasted. This wide spreading, magnificent tree is well honored in poems and a song for Christmas which recalls, "Chestnuts roasting on an open fire."

The Native People used dry Chestnut leaf tea as a medicine for whooping cough. There is a vaccination for whooping cough, but that was developed only recently. I had whooping cough as a young girl, and it is three months of serious illness. The resulting cough did sound like the whoop of some strange, large bird.

The recent decline of the Chestnut came with *Endothia parasitica*, a tiny parasite that attacked the inner bark of the Chestnut trees causing a fatal blight. Almost one fourth of the trees in the Eastern woodlands were Chestnuts, now there are very few left. There is research going on to find a blight resistant stock. The genetics of Chestnut (and many other plants) is complex. I hope it will allow the Chestnut to evolve into a tree that can withstand the blight without giving up its abundant nut crops. It would be a shame to lose such a wonderful gift of food and beauty.

We humans have learned to travel at great speed from one place in the world to another. I am afraid we often bring along parasites and insects that attack our trees and cause a lot of damage. In their point of origin, the trees of a place have been able to work up resistance to a parasite, so they are not destroyed. We are learning many things as we rearrange the world to suit our fancy. Many organisms that came down the newly opened St. Lawrence seaway and are having a field day reproducing in the waters of the Great Lakes. Sigh…perhaps that we can do something does not mean that we should do it.

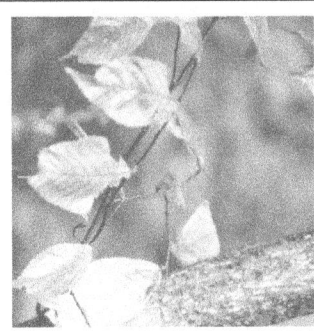

WOODS
Ostrya virginiana

Ironwood
(Hop Hornbeam)

Ironwood is an understory tree; it only grows twenty to forty feet tall. It is shade tolerant, deeply rooted and very slow growing. This tree keeps company with Oaks and Hickories. The name "Ironwood" says it all. The wood was used for sled runners, tool handles, yokes for oxen (very sturdy plow animals), wooden bowls and sometimes for bows. A swing with an ax is likely to bounce off this tree!

The outer bark is thin, light gray and shreddy, with loose narrow vertical strips that are turned out at the ends. The fruit is a cluster of papery sacs that form around the female flower. It looks like a "hops" bundle. These clusters are light green at first then turn brown in the autumn. The leaves are somewhat oval, doubly serrate, with long tapered points. Ironwood forms male and female catkins about the time the leaves are forming. The wind easily pollinates the tree before the leaves can block the motion of the air.

There are three layers of medicine in the bark of the Ironwood tree. The outer layer was prepared as a bark decoction (simmered for thirty minutes, then filtered) and the liquid was helpful as a blood builder and also for the aches of rheumatism. The inner bark (cambium layer) was also prepared as a decoction, but it was used for more serious conditions like high fever and to cleanse the blood from malaria attacks. We do not have many cases of malaria at the present time, but you can be sure the mosquitoes are still in existence waiting for us to take so many antibiotics that these medicines can no longer fight off disease. The bacteria continue to evolve, but they are faster than we are since they have short life cycles.

The heartwood of the tree could also be cooked and used as medicine for kidney pain, bad coughs, or bleeding in the lungs. The condition would need to be serious to take the life of the tree, whereas the medicinal bark could be stripped from smaller end branches leaving the tree to continue in this life cycle.

Ironwood is a sturdy tree. It sends down roots deep in the ground and tolerates most conditions that are part of a hardwood forest. But it cannot tolerate the salt we put on the roads. Salt is a problem for many trees and plants. The browning conifers along the road are an indication of too much salt and exhaust from cars.

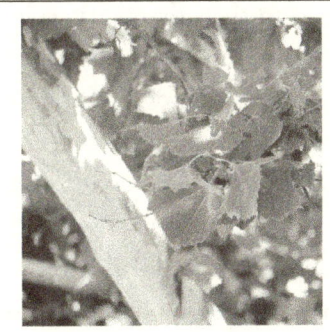

WOODS
Plantanus occidentalis

Sycamore

Sycamore is a fascinating tree. The outer bark is unusual. The upper tree bark is smooth, somewhat white but mottled with large patches of brown, green, and gray. At the base of the trunk, which can reach ten feet in diameter, the bark is dark brown and furrowed. This is a shade tree! The place of choice for Sycamore is the wet area near a river bank, lake, swamp, or a flood plain. It reminds me a bit of Weeping Willow in its shape and growth pattern

The leaves are somewhat Maple-shaped with pointed lobes. The male flowers grow in the angle where the twig joins the main branch. The female flowers grow at the ends of the twigs. All that is needed is a bit of wind for pollination. The fertilized flowers form round hanging balls that mostly stay on the tree for the winter. Sycamore needs moist sunny ground for its seeds to germinate.

Sycamore can live over five hundred years, long enough to outlive other trees in the neighborhood. It is not tolerant of other plants or grasses, the leaves produce an allelopathic herbicide that few other plants can tolerate. Sycamore wants and needs the benefit of full sunlight and wind.

Sycamore is a good friend to many animals. The leaves are very rich and make good worm beds. The old trees have cavities that make great den sites for possums, raccoons or owls. There was a time when the tree also gave homes to the chimney swifts (I suppose now they prefer chimneys). Wood ducks also use the Sycamore, as they nest above ground. When the young are big enough they tumble or half-fly from the tree to the nearest water to begin learning duck water skills.

As medicine, Sycamore has been used to treat dysentery, colds, coughs and the complications of measles. Old Sycamore stumps sprout into new growth which is a good source of twigs for inner bark to make a decoction.

The Sycamore is a good transition tree as we move from the woods to the wetlands. It can handle woodland conditions where there is enough moisture to meet the needs of such a large tree. A flood plain will also provide a good locale even though flooding occurs on an unpredictable schedule. The nearby water keeps the ground water level high enough to take care of this water loving tree.

WETLANDS

We move now to the places called wetlands. These wetlands may be the land around a pond, along the banks of a river, it may be a marsh or swamp or even a bog. Water is the central factor that provides a home-land just right for certain plants. All living beings, plants, and animals have cells that are sixty percent water, which shouldn't be a problem on a planet that is seventy percent water.

However, almost all the water is salt water. Fresh water is an endangered commodity which has its own cycle. The energy of the sun evaporates water from the oceans, lakes, rivers, ponds, plants leaves, even from the breath and bodies of animals. The water moves in clouds over the Earth. As this warm moist air cools it forms water droplets that fall on the land (it is fresh water now). Some of the rainwater evaporates again, some soaks into the ground into rock lined reservoirs that can flow like rivers. When a well is drilled, it is a reservoir that gives us water. As we make more people we need more water, sometimes more than rain can provide. Then we take too much from the ground and the earth collapses to fill the space—creating a sinkhole.

Here in the place of the Great Lakes we have an abundance of fresh water, except we seem determined to poison it! Factory runoff, mining liquids, all kinds of things are put into our drinking water. I believe we can clean up the Great Lakes if we care enough about the future of our children. This *sneaky stuff* worries me. Sometimes after a mine has been cleared of a metal resource, someone gets an idea that pouring a few million gallons of Sulfuric Acid into the hole will leach out more metal from a mine. The slightly used Sulfuric Acid will go either into the water of the Great Lakes, or into the ground to become part of the groundwater! Most of Wisconsin tilts to the South, anything put in the ground in northern Wisconsin will affect the water of the entire state. We need to protect this essential resource from pollution that can destroy our future.

I will speak now about the plants who have adapted themselves to life with their feet in the water. Wetland plants have evolved to deal with excess water. They absorb only what is needed and exclude the remaining water. This ability gives the plants a rich choice of nutrients for their use. My herb mother said the strongest medicines grow in wetlands.

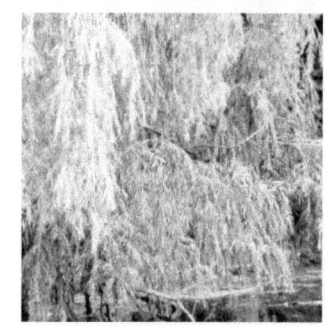

WETLANDS
Salix species

Willow

The Weeping **Willow** grows with her roots in the water. The smooth, slender, flexible branches hang over the water of the pond, almost as if she were looking at her own reflection. The People called her "Zasgomizh" which means "beautiful hair."

The color of the bark on these twigs changes through the seasons, from pale green in summer to a yellow gold in the color ceremony of autumn. A basket I made with a Red Osier frame ended up delightfully striped when the Willow twigs shifted their color. Yes, it took me a long time to weave. Such artistry is not my strong suit, but if I can do it, you can do it. Willow makes such pretty baskets.

The medicinal part of the Willow is the bark. The Willows have many small branches and are willing to share some as medicine. I put down an offering of Kinnik then tell the tree how the medicine will be used. I field strip the leaves at the tree so that their energy stays near the tree to be reabsorbed. The sticks I take to dry for medicine.

Willow bark contains an aspirin like compound called salicin, which is analgesic (stops pain) and styptic (stops bleeding). A mother drank tea made from Willow bark as part of the birthing process for the People. They believe a newborn should not hear screams of fear and pain at the moment of birth. Instead what is heard is the rhythm of a drum, beating the breathing rate of Life for mother and child. Some People used the bark of White Willow, some used the bark of Black Willow. I think it was determined by what tree happened to grow near the wigwams of the People.

This is the only pain reliever I learned from my herb mother. Pain is specific to what is causing the problem, so a headache required one kind of medicine, the ache of a broken bone needed another (or both, as pain is as simple or as complex as Life itself).

I want to talk a little about the responsibility of working with medicinal plants. This is where it gets tricky, as it is not my human efforts that create a cure. Since healing is mostly a gift from the Plants I cannot take money for medicine. When herbalists did all the doctoring, the People gifted food and such to them, so the herbalist would have time to gather and prepare medicines. This does not fit well into the present society, where that which is free is seen as being of no value. In this journal I talk about plants known to every family, so you may learn them, too.

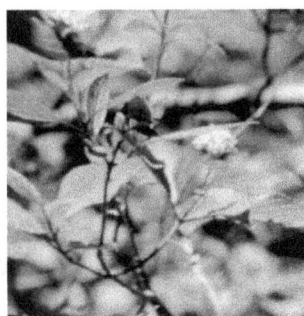

WETLANDS
Cornus stolonifera

Red Osier

This is a beautiful little tree. Its bark is shiny red and stays that way all year. *Cornus* seems to know it looks good even in the deep snows of winter. My grandmother called it a, "bend and stay" plant, as its flexible branches provided the frame for many baskets.

This plant was and is, very much a part of the lives of the People. Its taller Cornus relative is the tree that forms the frame of a wigwam. Seven trees are drawn together as rafters for a lodge. Each tree base is set into a hole which includes an offering of Kinnik. A gift of Kinnikinnik in the foundation of the wigwam frame is a thanksgiving to the Spirit of the Cornus which is now a part of their "Home." This reflects one of the philosophical guidelines for living of the People, the belief that "there will be enough for everyone if we only take what we truly need." This view of the world came from a People who knew "who they were, why they were here and how they fit in with all other Beings on the Earth."

Cornus is in the Dogwood Family, it grows up to ten feet tall. The leaves are oval with smooth margins, and the flowers are white and grow in flat topped clusters. Later in the season the flowers become clusters of white berries. The Evening Grosbeaks just love these berries. If they eat them after they have fermented the birds even get tipsy!

It is the bark that carries the medicinal gifting of this tree. My herb mother used the bark as a substitute for quinine when treating an intermittent fever. A bark decoction can also clear infected material from the intestines, making it a good helper to those with diverticulitis.

This tree has much to say in the way it welcomes animals, in the way it moves in the wind, in the way the light shimmers on the deep red branches. Be patient, as it is not such an easy thing for a plant to communicate. They do not use words (usually), so we need to listen in a way that they can be heard. I have seen little plants shimmer as if to get my attention. Some people dream about a plant, or feel good if they sit a near a certain kind of tree. The People watched the other animals when they had sickness, and noticed which plants these creatures chose. The other animals are older than we are, it serves us well to learn from these elders!

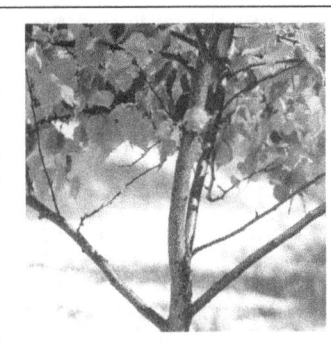

WETLANDS
Populus balsamifera

Balsam Poplar

Balsam Poplar has a number of common names like "Balm of Gilead" or its Indian name "Tacamahac," as it is called by the People of the East Coast. The early settlers had very little in the way of medicine, so this tree was a welcome gift. Young leaf buds cooked slowly in oil make a long-lasting salve which is anti-bacterial and helps with the pain of burns. The same oil mixture is a good liniment for sore muscles, sprains, rheumatism and backache. The buds contain methyl salicylate, an aspirin like compound which is released into the oil.

The dry buds prepared as a tea are very helpful for coughs and other lung problems, since it is an expectorant. It also helps with inflammation and promotes healing. The tree has not changed over the years, it still has these medicinal gifts to offer. I was delighted to find it growing along the shore of Lake Michigan, taking the opportunity to grow in places opened up to plant growth by the lowering of the Lake water. I do not know where that much water has gone, but the stone shelves give a history of many rises and falls in the Time before we came to "record" such changes.

Balsam Poplar likes wetlands near lakes, rivers or swamps. It grows quickly sometimes reaching sixty feet tall. Most do not reach that size, as they have shallow roots and tend to decay easily. The roots produce suckers—young trees to replace the fallen parent tree. The leaves are triangular with a flat base. The edges are coarse-toothed, fragrant and have a reddish color under the leaves. In looks and color this tree is very similar to the Birch. The People called this tree "Manasadi," which means "a kind of Aspen."

Some of the bark is thin and birch-like, but the young branches are dark coppery brown (at least some of them are). It can be a confusing identification unless you smell the leaf buds. They have a menthol fragrance to let you know this is "Tacamahac," the Balsam Poplar. The winter buds also have the medicine component and are there if you need the medicine during the cold months. The buds in an infusion are also a good poultice for frostbite; soak a clean cloth in the tea liquid and place the cloth gently on the affected skin. Perhaps it would be wiser to gather buds and make the salve before winter, but at least you know there is tree medicine that can help with cold hands, feet and faces.

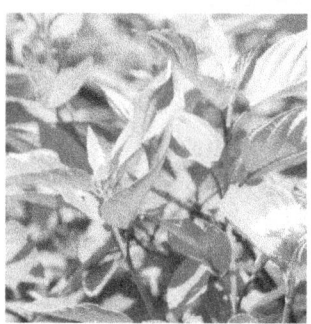

WETLANDS
Viburnum prunifolium

Blackhaw (Crampbark)

Blackhaw is a tall shrub, or a small tree, that grows up to thirty feet tall. I would call that a tree, but I am a short human. The leaves are oval with tiny toothed edges and the color is a dull green. The flowers are quite noticeable; white flowers in flat clusters. The berries form as a dark blue clump of shiny fruit that quickly turns black and shows up easily on the red stems. The Blackhaw prefers the low woodland areas. I suspect the extra ground moisture is helpful for fruit production.

This is a medicine tree. My herb mother used this medicine as a tonic for people. In general, it is a relaxant. It relaxes the peripheral blood vessels which helps lower blood pressure. More often she used the Blackhaw to prevent miscarriage. This medicine helps prevent spasms of the uterus. This is very helpful during the danger months early in pregnancy. She would stop using the Crampbark four weeks before the expected time of delivery.

My grandmother delivered over a hundred babies during her time as a midwife. There was a time not all that long ago, when cash first was the only way for an Indian to be admitted to a hospital. Someone had to deliver the babies. The cambium bark (the inner layer below the protective outer covering) is the way to utilize the gift of this tree. A few short branches will provide all the cambium usually needed and the herbalist can offer Kinnik in thanksgiving knowing the tree is not harmed by the small gathering. Two teaspoons of cambium bark simmered for ten minutes in a pint of water is the best and easiest method with Crampbark. A tablespoon, morning and evening, is the dosage to begin with.

Blackhaw is anti-spasmodic which also makes it helpful for asthma. It is also anti-inflammatory, as it contains salicin like Willows do. Blackhaw is gentle enough to be a tonic. This is important for chronic conditions that require medication over a longer period of time. With conditions that end in "itis," like arthritis, a pain relieving tonic can help the body with disease and perhaps even help a damaged immune system remember how to work properly.

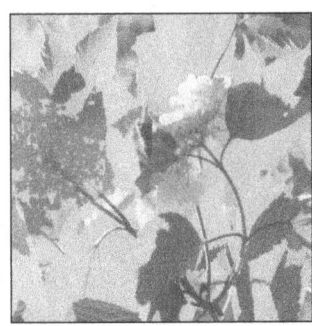

WETLANDS
Viburnum opulus

Highbush Cranberry

This *Viburnum* is a shrub tree, and it grows under taller trees reaching to about ten feet tall. I have found it growing on the upslope of a swale (the wet area beyond the shore that gets occasional flood water). This tree is also called Crampbark, as the bark is anti-spasmodic. I use the cambium bark from the end twigs to make a decoction. The tree can spare some of these twigs and I do not harm the life cycle of this helpful medicine tree. Two teaspoons of shaved bark simmered in a pint of water is enough medicine for a day.

Whenever possible it is best to make the medicine fresh each day, that way none of the potency is lost and there is no concern about it spoiling. Plant medicines leave plant proteins in the water, and these proteins begin to break down within a day of shelf time. Plant medicine is good but it is also tempting to over eager molds.

A Viburnum bark decoction is used for asthma, or for convulsions. An infusion (boiling water poured over bark and steeped for ten minutes) is strong enough for muscle spasms or menstrual cramps.

Highbush Cranberry has gray bark and leaves shaped like Maple leaves. If you look underneath the maple-like leaves you will find that the Viburnum leaves are hairy. The flowers are white and they form good sized round blossoms up to four inches across. As the season progresses the blossoms are replaced by bright red berries that may stay on the tree all winter. The People called this tree "Aniibimin," which is "Elm berry." The berries are high in Vitamin C and Vitamin K. The People did not use the word "vitamin" but they were aware that a tea from the berries could keep them healthy through the long winter. The berries are a bit high in acid, like cranberries, and may need honey or maple syrup to sweeten the tea.

A tea made from Viburnum berries and a little bark might be very helpful for someone who cannot relax when it is time to sleep. This is not a sleeping potion, but a tea that lets the muscles relax and calms the nerves. Perhaps it neutralizes the excess adrenaline still running through the body, I don't know for sure, but it does help the muscles to relax.

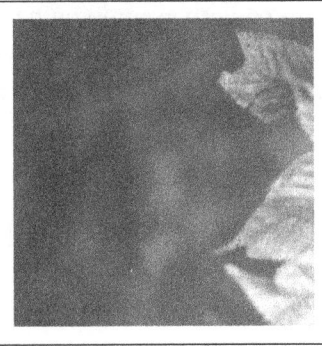

WETLANDS
Larix laricina

Tamarack

The word for medicine, "Mashki," is the same as the word for "Swamp" in the language of the People. This is the next part of our plant journey. I hope you are wearing your expendable sneakers, as this is a dark, rich, organic place, with lots of water. This is still water, as it is not moved by wind or river current. This swamp place is quiet, and the surrounding trees seem to absorb all unnecessary sound. I always put down tobacco before going into this place.

We could call this place a "Tamarack Swamp," many of the trees are Tamaracks. "Mashki Gwaatig" is the name for this tree, it means "Medicine Tree," which it truly is. In summer the needles of this tree are a pale blue-green color, and grow in clusters along the branches. This conifer is deciduous, meaning that in autumn the needles turn a gold color and fall off the tree. The fallen needles leave distinctive empty nodes along the branches. Tamarack has a shallow root system and falls over easily. The fallen tree makes good shelter for the snowshoe hares that live in these places.

Tamarack is my favorite tree. The pitch of this tree can be used whenever conifer sap is needed in a recipe. The inner bark is medicinal and it makes a good poultice for a wound. In a decoction this inner bark is alterative, meaning it will bring about a change in a stubborn condition! The cambium bark is anti-inflammatory and acts as a kidney nudge where there are signs of jaundice (yellowing of the skin).

This is a "be careful" medicine tree. It is easy to make the medicine too strong. Learning the ways of medicine takes a lot of time, but it is part of my responsibility to the safety of the People. I do not usually work with plants that are listed as heavily toxic, or poisonous.

Tamarack is a good tree to get acquainted with even if you have no need of its particular medicine. The short needles are very soft, like little paint brushes. It also has little cones, about half an inch long, that are a lovely mahogany color and look almost varnished.

A swamp or bog is very high in tannin, and there are very few bacteria that can live in the acidity of the place. Tannins and other minerals leach out of the fallen trees. They are absorbed by other plants growing in the area and become a part of their medicinal sharing (nothing is wasted).

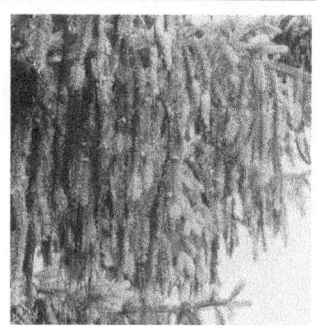

WETLANDS
Picea mariana

Black Spruce

Black Spruce chooses the wetlands. It is a familiar sight in the northern swamps. This Spruce can tolerate the water, but it cannot tolerate fire. Black Spruce will grow in stands of itself, or share space with Cedars, Tamaracks and Balsam Fir trees. It is an indicator tree for water near the surface of the ground (your basement will leak!).

Black Spruce is not a tall tree (usually), maybe reaching forty feet tall in a good growing location. It can live a long life, up to two hundred years. This is not a pretty tree, as it has "open spots" where branches have fallen and the older branches droop. Even when the lower branches die they do not always fall off, this gives the tree a "scraggly" appearance. The trunk bark is grayish brown and has scaly, resin-sticky bark. This pitch forms thick clumps where the tree has been injured. This easy-to-gather pitch is sold as "Spruce gum," in case you wondered where it came from.

The needles are about a half inch long, rather stiff and pointy. They grow out of all sides of the branches. These needles can live up to seven years before falling out leaving little woody knolls somewhat like the Tamarack nodes. This Spruce has a nice fragrance, the needles carry a fresh resin smell that is very nice.

The Black Spruce is shallow rooted, and the rootlets run close to the surface of the ground. This does not give the tree a solid foundation, perhaps another reason this tree chose the protected areas of the wetlands.

The People used the long slender roots of Black Spruce for fine lacing. They called the roots "wattup" and were very grateful for this gift of Black Spruce. In a very harsh winter the needles and bark from small twigs could be boiled into a tea to prevent scurvy. They would drink this tea every other day, as there is too much tannin to consider it a pleasant daily beverage. The People did not use the word "scurvy" (and there was no word for vitamin C), but all the Native Peoples knew how to cure the sickness. The inner bark of Black Spruce worked as a poultice for infection in a cut or wound. The People of the Great Lakes were taught many medicines to preserve their health, fortunately for early colonists, the Native People were willing to share this knowledge.

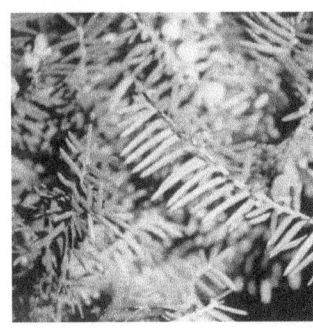

WETLANDS
Taxus canadensis

Yew

Yew is a shrub growing with no particular shape, but surrounding itself with others of its kind. The flat needles have tiny stalks, and appear to be pointed at both ends. They look a lot like Fir needles, with tiny white stripes underneath. The Yew is browse for both deer and moose. Otherwise most animals find the Yew thickets a good nursery or hiding place for their young.

Yew has worthy defenses, as it produces hormones in the leaves that can stop the life cycle of insect predators. It produces a bright red berry-like aril (fruit pod that is shaped like a bell), which can be safely eaten by hungry birds. For humans the story is different, as the aril contains taxine, which is deadly poison. One aril can kill a child. I don't know why we plant such poisonous plants as ornamental bushes for our homes, or near the schools!

In America and in Europe the wood of the Yew has been used for making bows. It is a resilient wood which sends an arrow on its way with accuracy and speed. Yew also gave wood for the making of trigger traps, which were used to capture small game animals.

The Native People did not domesticate animals, because their meat supply was whatever the forest offered—Moose, Elk, Deer, Porcupine, Muskrat, Rabbit and many other animal beings all gave themselves as food for a hungry People. The hunters spoke to the animals and thanked them for their offering. It was part of the balance that no species be hunted to the point of being endangered.

It is a mystery of medicine that the sap from the bark of the Yew, once used to poison the tips of arrows, is now being researched as a way to treat breast and ovarian cancer. It is not that a tree is good or bad, but we need to find a relationship with the tree that respects our Spirit and the Spirit of the tree. My herb mother would be proud that Western Medicine has begun to research plants and trees growing in our own country. The tricky part is not to research the plant or tree into early extinction.

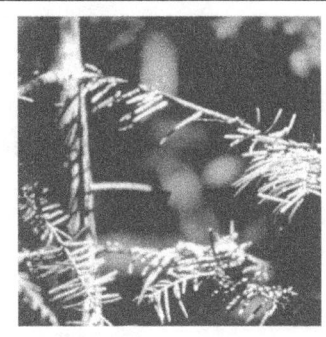

WETLANDS
Abies balsamea

Balsam Fir

This is the evergreen called "Elder Sister" by the People. Her longer name, "Nimissay" means "she speaks for us." My grandmother said, "If you are in difficulty and your hands are not free to say a prayer, then ask Elder Sister to send your prayer to the Great Spirit." The top of the **Balsam Fir** is peaked, something like the spire at the top of a Church.

Balsam Fir needles are flattened and very aromatic. There are two parallel white lines on the under side of the needles. The bark is ash gray and smooth, with pitch blisters along the trunk of the tree. The cones stand upright on the branches like candles!

There was a time when specimen slides for microscope viewing were coated with Balsam Fir sap to keep out air. This was an adaptation of the main spiritual gifting of this tree. The sap that forms in the blisters is antiseptic, analgesic and forms an airtight covering. This is perfect for burns. There is a very brief time before the pain of a serious burn begins. If the burn area is covered quickly with Balsam sap this pain does not happen! Okay, the pitch is a bit sticky. I put a coating of baby powder on the outer surface so the person doesn't stick to everything.

To gather Balsam Fir sap you need only a safety pin and a small jar. Ask the tree for sap, put down an offering, then poke a tiny hole in the bottom of the pitch blister. Carefully press down on the blister and the sap will ooze out of the hole into the jar. After a couple of blisters you won't need to worry about dropping the pin, it is attached to your fingers with sap! If you are patient and work a few hours you may be able to collect half an ounce. Collecting sap this way is a bit like milking a mosquito, but you will surely enjoy this hobby.

Herbalism is a labor of love, but this sap is a wonderful gift for people who get burned. I make the smallest possible hole in the tree bark so the tree can close up and keep out fungus or mold. I believe it is a part of our responsibility to the Balsam Fir to see to its health for the future. You know where it leads when we humans decide that we can take whatever we want from the Planet. Simply put, plants do not need us but we need plants to survive.

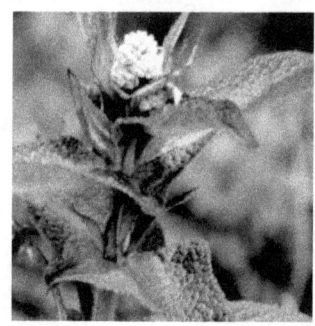

WETLANDS
Eupatorium perfoliatum

Boneset

Boneset is an appropriate common name for this wetland plant. It is a perennial, growing from rhizomes which allow colonies of the plant to form. The flowers are usually white in flat clusters at the top. Perhaps you think that all the plants look alike! Not Boneset. Look at the leaves, they are opposite, and it looks like the stem is inserted through the middle of the connected leaf pairs. My grandmother called it "shield and lance" plant. If that doesn't help, the leaves are very wrinkled like an elderly plant. It is also a very hairy plant, as the top and bottom of the leaves and even the stems have lots of hair.

Late in the summer when the Boneset is finished with its flowering, I go out to gather leaves. Boneset helps the body with the "aches of influenza." I use it with Catnip since it is usually a low fever that causes this condition. The body is clever, as it will get sick to stop us from being busy and to let the body rest and recover its balance. Boneset also helps clear mucus from the upper respiratory tract.

The common cold is a year-round phenomenon, so I need to gather enough dry leaves to last the entire year.

The primary Spiritual gift of Boneset is to mend the sclerotic lining of bones when there is a crack or a break. This is perfect for elders who sometimes break a hip and they can't seem to heal. The lining of the bone must be mended and that is what Boneset will do. It lowers the risk of "bone fever" which is an infection within the bone. Often I give Boneset to people who slip on the ice and crack a rib. This plant cuts the healing time in half. Usually all the doctors can do for cracked ribs is to tape the area (sometimes), and tell you not to cough or sneeze.

Boneset tea is not tasty, it doesn't even pretend to be! Most people would rather have the pain than drink this tea, as it has an "earthy" taste. The Boneset leaves crumble easily and will powder in a coffee mill. It is much easier to get someone to take gelatin capsules. It is perhaps not the best way, but it will work. I have people take eight capsules a day.

Perhaps I should talk more about the sclerotic lining. This is also what covers the eyes, the heart and other inner organs of the body. I have given Boneset to someone who scratched their eye. With children, the Boneset powder can be mixed in with applesauce. Half the challenge of herbalism is figuring out how to get the medicine inside the human.

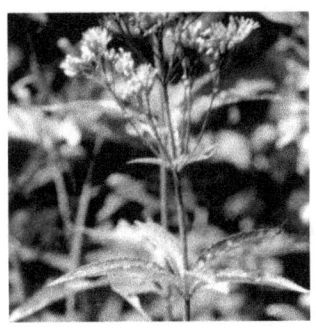

WETLANDS
Eupatorium purpureum

Joe Pye Weed

This other "Eupatoium cousin" also grows with its feet in water. It is tall, up to six feet, and it also has a root and rhizome system which founds colonies of this wetland plant. The blossoms are large rounded clusters of pink or purple flowers at the top of the plant. The leaves are toothed and grow in well spaced whorls along the stem. The stem is green with noticeable black splotches at the leaf joints. The leaves have a mild vanilla fragrance.

During the time of colonization there was an Abenaki medicine man named Zhopai who lived near Stockbridge, Massachusetts. During an epidemic of flu and fever this medicine man treated the family of a white blacksmith who was his friend. The next year when the Stockbridge People moved to Wisconsin, Zhopai was left behind, because he had done too many favors for whites. Zhopai gave his grandchildren seeds from the *Eupatorium* to plant along their migration path so that this medicine plant would always be there. Joe Pye now grows as far West as Wisconsin.

I gather leaves every summer after the plant has blossomed. The leaves are big, so I can take a few from many plants and not interfere with their autumn cycle. A tea from Joe Pye leaves is still good medicine for flu. The leaves contain polysaccharides which are a boost to the immune system. The tea also helps the body work against the fever and pains of influenza...a good plant.

Sometimes I also gather the roots of this plant. The roots are strong medicine, they are diuretic, antilithic (stones), and antirheumatic. The healing gift of this root is to dissolve stones which form in the kidneys or gall bladder. Joe Pye certainly deserves the offering of Kinnik, it is amazing!

If there is a family tendency to kidney or gall stones, Joe Pye root can be a fine preventive tonic. Stones hurt, so it is much better to avoid the painful journey by dissolving them. In the mystery that is our body, this tonic can also help with certain kinds of arthritis as well. To make the root tonic, add one teaspoon of chopped root to one cup of cold water. Heat and simmer in a covered kettle for fifteen minutes. Pour the liquid through a filtering cloth and it is ready to drink (add honey if you wish). One cup a day is enough as a preventive.

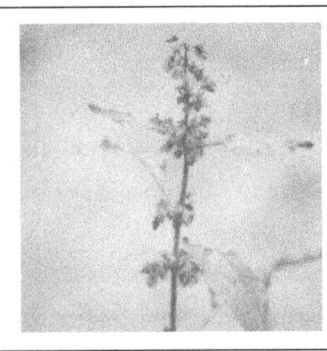

WETLANDS
Scutellaria lateriflora

Marsh Skullcap

This is a perennial wetland Mint. It grows to about eighteen inches tall on a rather weak square stem. The leaves are opposite, oval and bluntly toothed. **Marsh Skullcap** has little bluish-purple hooded flowers growing from the leaf axils.

True to its common name, Marsh Skullcap grows in the marsh, wet meadows, or along the low banks of a river. Marsh Skullcap has a root/rhizome so there will be a number of plants in a given area.

The medicinal gift comes from the above ground parts which are best gathered early in the summer. A teaspoon of dry plant to a cup of boiling water is the best way to release the medicinal aspect. Marsh Skullcap is sedative, nervine and anti-spasmodic. It is helpful for insomnia, neuralgia and nervous irritation (twitches). There was a time when it was also used to help with convulsions and epilepsy. It is an indication that the gift of this plant is consistent; it helps a person relax.

Chemically the plant contains scutellarin, which is a flavonoid compound that acts as a sedative and is anti-spasmodic. Flavonoids are being researched now. Flavonoid glycosides (which is the way they come in plants) are chemicals found in living plant tissue. They are found in the flowers, fruit and leaves of certain plants. Plants with white and yellow flowers seem to have the highest levels of flavonoids, plants like Yarrow, Elder and Lime (Basswood). The flavonoids in the flowers appear to attract pollinating insects. However, they are also toxic to certain other insects and defend the plant from these insect predators.

Active Flavonoid compounds are diuretic, anti-inflammatory, antiseptic and sometimes even anti-tumor. They usually affect the vascular system and are very helpful for circulatory problems. Using the vascular system allows the compounds to travel to all areas where their help might be needed. The medicine is transported to all affected joints to help with arthritis.

Sharing compounds is balanced help. These flavonoids defend the Marsh Skullcap and help with reproduction. In our bodies they can bring relief from inflammatory problems, high blood pressure, restlessness and other conditions.

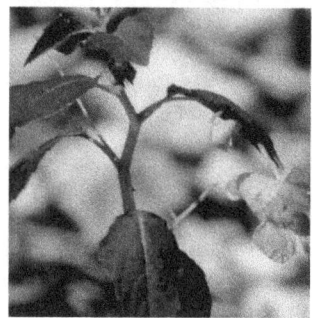

WETLANDS
Impatiens biflora

Jewelweed

I begin with a teaching story. "Frog hopped away from the pond to sing his love song. He was so busy with courtship matters that he didn't notice Snake until it was almost too late. Snake was sure he'd have a meal. At the last possible moment, Frog leaped into a huge bed of Poison Ivy! Snake knew he didn't want that itchy rash the full length of his belly, so he didn't go after Frog. He merely hissed a wish that Frog would be all itchy, and that would serve Frog right for not staying around to be eaten. Frog was very clever, he waited until Snake was gone, then hopped into a patch of **Jewelweed** plants. Frog rolled on the plants and rubbed himself all over with the stem juice of this helpful plant. It was good for Frog to know this plant, and it will do the same for people."

Rhus radicans, which we call Poison Ivy, is amazingly persistent. It is long lived and can clone itself into huge colonies. It can grow in any kind of soil, but it loves the limey soil of the Great Lakes! Poison

Ivy has two forms; it can be a low shrub or it can be a climbing vine. It will grow in the sun or in the shade. Poison Ivy leaflets may be toothed or smooth, they may be rounded or pointed, and these changeable leaves may even be shiny or dull! The only constant is it has three leaflets.

The Poison Ivy plant contains an oily sap. A chemical in the sap causes an allergic reaction in humans (no fur). Some people show immunity to Poison Ivy but this can change very suddenly. It is better to treat this plant with great respect (it just doesn't like people)!

My herb mother said the antidote to a toxic plant will always grow nearby, if we only have the wisdom to know what it is. I have used fresh Jewelweed plant when I have accidentally walked into Poison Ivy, and it works! Jewelweed has long, translucent stems which are thick at the joints and very juicy. It is this inner liquid which has the healing gift of the plant.

This liquid is antidote for most plant rashes, including Nettle, Algae and most Fungal rashes. This is a fun medicinal to make. I gather long pieces of Jewelweed stem, cut them into two inch lengths, then pound them with a rock. Bruising helps the stem juice leach out. I put the pieces of stem into a canning jar, tightly packed, then fill the jar with rubbing alcohol. The alcohol turns orange after a couple weeks of shaking. When filtered it is good medicine for any mysterious rash.

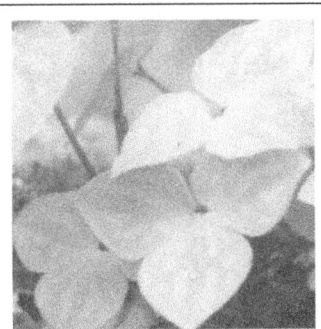

WETLANDS
Hepatica americana

Liverwort

I cannot called this plant **Liverwort**. The word Hepatica is a better honoring for the plant. *Hepatica* is an evergreen perennial with a fascinating life cycle. It is an early Spring plant, and can send up a flower before the snow is melted. Sometimes there are no leaves, just the flower, which can be white, pink, or blue depending on the species of Hepatica. Without the distinctive lobed leaves, an early hiker may wonder what plant this is (I have). Surprisingly there are little flies and some brave early bees who will see to the pollination.

There is the round leaf Hepatica that prefers acidic soil, the sharp leaf Hepatica that chooses limey soil. There may be both in the same place, or they may hybridize to please themselves. The leaves also have this kind of whimsy. Older leaves sometimes have a purplish color, or there may be the three lobed new green leaf to go with the flower. Not surprising the flower also has choices about how many petals to have, usually between six and ten petals.

Hepatica can also grow happily in Maple forests. They are comfortable with shade although they utilize the early Spring sunlight for flower making. The Maples have not yet leafed out when the Hepatica flowers. This is a small plant, only about four inches tall. It has a hairy stem, perhaps for protection against the cold temperature.

Medicinally Hepatica is as uncertain as its other aspects. *Hepatica* belongs to the Buttercup family and most of these plants are toxic. I hope there is research being done on this plant, as it may have help to share for Lupus or other serious liver problems. I do not know and am not willing to experiment with it on someone who already has a weakened state of health. So I see the Hepatica in the early Spring and give thanks for the beauty which it shares with those who walk the woodlands and the wetlands.

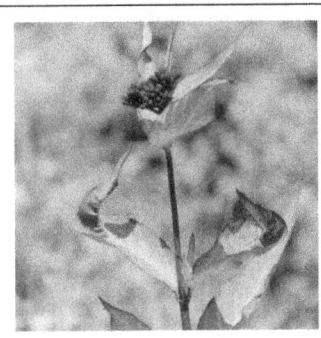

WETLANDS
Asclepias incarnata

Swamp Milkweed

The **Milkweed** Family, *Asclepiadaceae*, are the milky juice plants. The white liquid, which contains potent toxins is mostly to defend the plants from insect feeders. The leaves are large and somewhat waxy and the flowers are five parted (the perfect flowers, so the botanists say). The petals of the blossoms are turned back out of the way at the time of pollination. The stamins and pistils are easily found by the bees and butterflies. The pollen is thick and waxy and often clumps on the legs of the bee. Sometimes the pollen load is so thick and heavy, the bee is killed while tangled in the blossoms.

Swamp Milkweed is well named, as it chooses the open, sunny places of swamps or river edges. This Milkweed grows about three feet tall and is a slender version of its dry field cousin. The flowers are deep pink, branched, flat topped clusters. The leaves are narrow, lance-shaped, and attached to the main stem by very short stems. The leaves are somewhat soft and are hairy on their undersides. The seed pods also are long and slender, although the seeds and "silken" parachutes are similar to the field Milkweed. It is this swamp version that makes the best cordage. The Native Americans used the spun thread for small animal traps and the netting part of the fish "weirs" (traps).

The roots of Swamp Milkweed are toxic if taken internally (causing violent vomiting). However, this same root infusion is an excellent soak for a swollen arm or leg. It is a quick diuretic to draw out the fluid buildup from injury or inflammation. For a People who walked from one place to another, and ate the food which they grew or gathered, the use of arms and legs was very important.

The way of medicine today is more likely to apply ice to keep down swelling. This works well if you have ice. Ice is not always a choice and somehow I wonder if the plant itself contains other healing gifts that just aren't found in ice cubes.

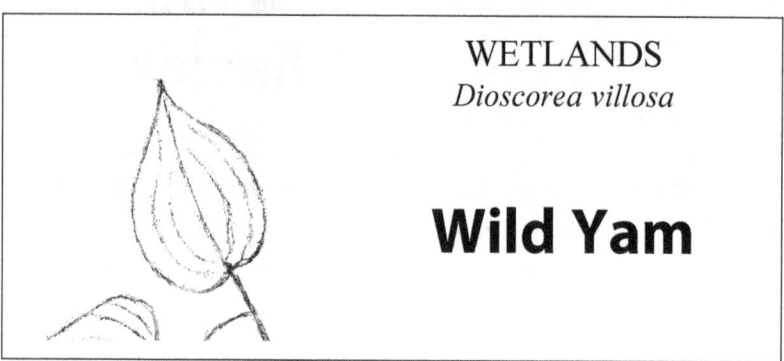

WETLANDS
Dioscorea villosa

Wild Yam

Wild Yam is a perennial twining vine with a smooth stem. It wraps around other handy plants and lets sunlight soak into leaves that are smooth on top and hairy underneath. These leaves are heart shaped with noticeable pronounced veins. The flowers and resulting seed pods are small but multiple on slender stems branching out from the main stem to allow for pollination.

One of the earliest medical uses of the root was as an anti-spasmodic for cramps or colic. This anti-spasmodic effect also offers help for migraine headaches (arterial spasms) and some types of high blood pressure. Wild Yam even offers some help for epilepsy (seizures) and spasmodic coughs. It is wise to avoid this plant during pregnancy since the birth process requires strong muscle contractions.

Wild Yam contains Diosgenin which is a plant steroid. This means the plant is also anti-inflammatory and anti-rheumatic. As medical research laboratories coax the cortisones and hydrocortisones from the Wild Yam plant tissue, the resulting medicine may offer symptom relief for allergies, bursitis, rheumatoid arthritis (especially at times of high inflammation) and also sciatica.

There have been topical creams made from Wild Yam root that promise to balance the hormone levels during a difficult menopause.

But a plant steroid is not the same as a human steroid; it works for plants to meet the need of the living plant. Most plant compounds either protect a plant from predators or attract a pollinator. Without the assistance of a chemical lab this expensive cream is probably most likely to help only with insect bites or rheumatism pain.

The hormonal changes of menopause are not all that different from the challenges of puberty. The hormone levels fluctuate (sometimes a lot) and make it a noticeable time. When a person has the flu or a cold, they say "I do not feel well." This is the same for unpredictable shifts of internal chemistry. Eventually the body restores the balance, and a level of hormones is established to maintain the body after the potential child bearing years. There are ways to help with the journey but expensive creams are probably not the answer.

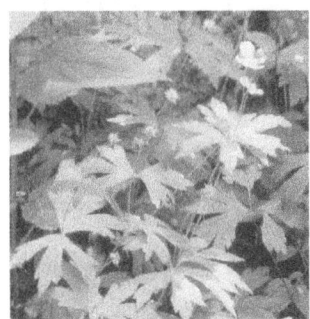

WETLANDS
Anemone canadensis

Canada Anemone

This plant grows in large patches in a wet meadow. **Canada Anemone** is perennial, grows to about two feet tall, and moves with the wind "dancing" with others of its kind. The basal leaves have long stalks. The upper leaves hold directly to the stalk without any stem. The flowers are white with five sepals up to an inch long.

If you happen to find this plant, spend some time watching and listening. The People called this plant "Midewidjibik," which means "Medicine Root." Canada Anemone is one of the plants taken into the Medicine Lodge to help with healing. The healing is as much spiritual as it is physical. Sometimes people get deeply attached to their illness and it is difficult for them to heal. I know this sounds peculiar and yet there are so many chronic conditions that get a hold of people. We lose a lot of good energy to the pain of arthritis, rheumatism and the other "isms" that plague our species. Perhaps the Spirit of Canada Anemone might help with this difficulty. It wouldn't hurt to ask.

The leaves of Canada Anemone are astringent, styptic, and antiseptic. It is a good poultice for a cut or scrape since it will kill germs as well as stopping the bleeding. The Native Americans used it specifically for nosebleeds.

The root can also be used in an infusion. Cooled water which carries the healing energy of Canada Anemone is a good soaking medium for the aches of rheumatism and the loss of fine motor skills that are part of this problem. I have not found a large patch of this plant. Perhaps it might also help with paralysis or loss of motion, but I have not found enough of this plant to test it.

Canada Anemone belongs to the Buttercup family which is always caustic and sometimes is toxic. The safest way to test a plant from this family is to try a small amount to see if there are negative affects. But I do not even do this until I have spoken to the plant to see if it is agreeable to helping people. (I ask carefully and respectfully as some plants do not like people). Like Poison Ivy, it doesn't bother other animals, just people. Even if the plant does not offer its medicine, it is still beautiful and may want to help in some other way.

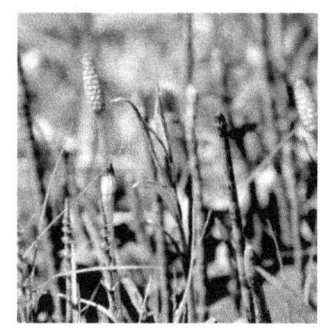

WETLANDS
Equisetum arvense

Horsetails

This plant looks its age, as it is a remnant of the age of the dinosaurs. It has a stiff, rough textured stem and branches without any apparent leaves. The nodes of the stem have teeth, which are really the leaves of this plant. It has different forms depending on what sort of reproductive mood the plant is in. The sterile shafts have stiff branchlets growing out and up from the nodes along the stem. It looks a bit like a stiff little Christmas tree. In this form the plant has the nickname "shavegrass." The fertile stems, called "horsetails," have a spore cap at the top supported by a single upright stem.

Equisetum has a high silica content, the main ingredient in sand. The People gathered both forms of this plant to use as sand paper for arrow shafts and other surfaces that needed smoothing. My herb mother did not want this plant used as a medicinal.

There is a Nanabooshoo story that tells a little of the history of this plant: "Once, long ago, Nanabooshoo went on a rampage. He rearranged lakes, pulled up mountains and blew out a lot of sand dunes. Some People thought it was delightful, especially if they had wanted a pathway to somewhere. Others thought it was terrible. They had just gotten used to where things were, and someone moved it all around.

Nanabooshoo was tired after all this and lay down to sleep for a long time. When he finally woke up something was holding him down! Finally he lay still and heard singing, "Ah ee, woe is me." "Who is singing," Nanabooshoo asked. A tiny voice answered, "I am, I'm the one holding you down. I have seen you go around thinking you are so important, you better hear my story."

"Once I was the tallest most handsome tree on the Earth. I knew I was the best of all Creation, I didn't want other creatures to interfere with my beauty. I wouldn't let vines climb my trunk, or insects walk on me. I surely wouldn't let birds make their dirty nests in my branches. I was so busy admiring myself I didn't notice I was getting smaller and smaller. Now here I am a tiny little plant!" Nanabooshoo had listened because he was held down, "I still don't see that a tiny plant like you can do anything to help a great spirit like me!" Nanabooshoo certainly didn't learn humility even though he had to listen to the plant.

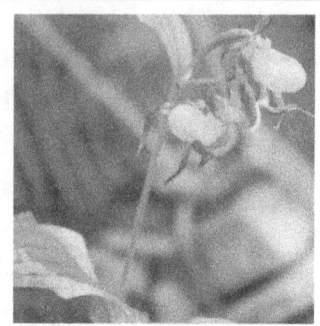

WETLANDS
Cypripedium calceolus

Ladyslipper

Ladyslipper is a beautiful, primitive member of the Orchid Family. It is rare now so I do not gather it, but a Ladyslipper is a joy to find and admire. The Native People called it "Makasin," which means "Moccasin Plant." It does indeed look like the puckered toe moccasins of the Great Lakes Indians. Ladyslipper prefers limestone areas and happily grows in old deer yards hidden away in Cedar swamps where the soil is loose and aerated. It will also be found in wet woods, along wooded shorelines, and near bogs and swamps.

The yellow Ladyslipper has long, stemless, folded leaves. The leaves have parallel veining and are pale and hairy underneath. There are fifty species of Ladyslippers, eleven of them found in North America. This Ladyslipper is easy to identify when it is flowering. There is a large, beautiful yellow pouch which sometimes has colorful stripes along the pathway it has chosen for pollinators. The nectar hairs lead the insect to a sticky receptacle inside the flower sac. To leave the flower the insect must travel a narrow path, touching the antlers as it goes, coating itself with pollen to take to the next flower. Sometimes the insect gets trapped inside the flower, and you'll find "chew holes" in the side of the flower pouch where an impatient bee has bitten its way out!

Ladyslipper has tuberous roots with thready fibers that spread out to form next years plants. A colony of these beautiful flowers is not unusual. The plant produces tiny winged seeds that travel on the wind. There is no food on the seeds, so they must land where there are mycorrhyzal fungi to provide food for the new plants. It can take two years for the seeds to germinate. These difficulties are part of the reason the Ladyslipper is rare.

When the forests and swamps were undisturbed, the People of the Great Lakes used the root of this plant as medicine. They found it helpful for nerve disorders and for migraine headaches. Migraines can also be treated with Pearly Everlasting, so the Ladyslipper can continue its life cycle undisturbed by a needy herbalist! In fact, touching the plant sometimes gives humans a rash. I am willing to accept the gift of beauty and realize some plants are there to please themselves with a life cycle that does better without interference.

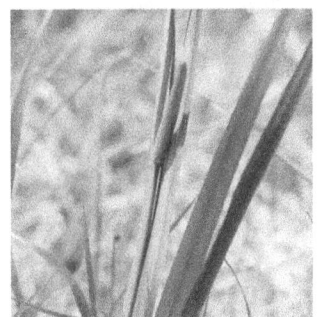

WETLANDS
Acorus calamus

Sweetflag

In a wet meadow or at the edge of a pond or river, sometimes tucked in among a grouping of Cattails, you may find Calamus. The first time I found Calamus was along a small river in New York. It was the fragrance of the plant that gave it away. It looks like a short Cattail plant but the root gives off an aromatic sweetness. We moved aside some rich black soil and there was the bright orange root. Actually the roots (rhizomes) join the Calamus plants into a colony. The roots we collected were about the diameter of my little finger. We harvested sections of root between some of the plants then carefully closed over the roots to continue the life cycle. This past summer, about fifteen years after the first meeting, I found Calamus plants, this time they were in flower. The flowers are tiny little yellow-green blossoms on a club-like flower stem called a spadix.

Calamus has a strong spirit for healing. I have put the fresh root into a tincture to soak out some of the gift of this plant. In small doses (a little nibble of fresh root), it treats the symptoms of sore throat. When I need to talk and sing on the same day, I keep a small piece of root in my mouth and my voice does not give out. Native singers also chew the root so they can sing all the songs the People want to hear (and dance to).

Calamus has mucilage, volatile oil, glycosides and tannins (a small piece is plenty to chew). Medically it is carminative (settles upset stomach), demulcent (soothing to inflamed tissue), and antispasmodic (especially for a frequent, dry cough). For a cold or cough, the chopped root can be prepared as an infusion. I often put some Calamus in with Mullein to make a cough syrup. The Calamus is good for any kind of gastric upset (it is a "bitter" which helps with digestion). It is also helpful for heartburn.

Calamus inhibits the growth of certain bacteria. This is good for sore throat as otherwise germs multiply in that warm, wet environment. It is also possible that Calamus helps lower serum cholesterol. If so, this is a very fine gift. When a plant is this helpful it is important not to over-harvest in the wild. Herb companies grow their own stock of Calamus and are there to provide the root if you need it. Our best conservation comes from knowing how important these plants are, both to themselves and to us.

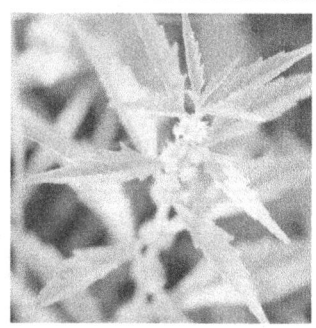

WETLANDS
Lycopus americana

Bugleweed

Bugleweed is a perennial mint whose height matches its surroundings, from six inches to three feet tall. There is no advantage for some plants in being the tallest if they have to fight the wind to stay upright. Bugleweed is very clever, as it has lance-shaped lower leaves with long narrow bases. The wide part of the leaf is outermost where it can capture the sunlight. It has the typical square stem of a Mint, and flowers that grow in the leaf axils.

In the same wet places is a plant of the same genus (*Lycopus*), it has the common name of Water Horehound. It also has opposite leaves with jagged edges, and tubular flowers in the leaf axils. These two cousins are almost interchangeable in their medical gifting. Water Horehound specializes in assisting the lungs, and has been used for coughs, consumption and bleeding of the lungs. As a leaf tea, which doesn't even taste bad, it is also hypoglycemic. Hypoglycemia is a fluctuation of blood sugar with periodic loss of energy throughout the day.

Bugleweed specializes in heart problems, especially a rapid pulse (palpitations). It is also very good for coughs and chronic lung problems. In times of food shortage the People would harvest the roots, dry them, then boil and eat them. (What is "food" changes with how hungry a person is.) In today's world people still starve to death. It is not the worst idea to know what can or cannot be eaten.

Both these plants are tonic to the thyroid gland. They help to balance the hormones that regulate metabolism. Metabolism is the conversion of food sugars to energy. Low metabolism results in overweight people with very little available energy. High metabolism results in very thin people who use up their energy too quickly. What the body needs is to find the balance that allows enough energy to do what needs to be done in life.

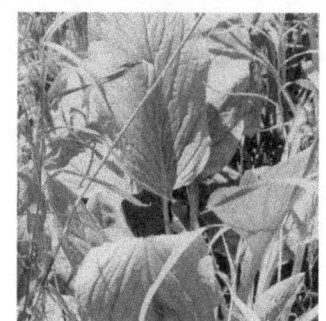

WETLANDS
Symplocarpus foetidus

Skunk Cabbage

Even the Latin name of this plant, *foetidus*, suggests the most noticeable aspect of this plant, which refers to the smell of something rotten. The Indian name "Zhigaagobag," means "Skunk Plant." There was a place in Illinois where there were many **Skunk Cabbage** plants growing, and the People of the Great Lakes called it "Zhigaago" (Chicago). Farther North along the shore of Lake Michigan, was another place which would become a city. It was called "Mzilaukee" which means "fertile Earth." Over time the name would slip over to its present form, Milwaukee. My grandmother heard about these places from her grandmother. She was disappointed to see what had happened to these beautiful places.

Skunk Cabbage grows in swamps, bogs, wet woodlands, and along the banks of rivers. The flower emerges early in the Spring. The respiration of the plant melts the snow around it and up comes a reddish-brown hood covering a fertile spathe. The fetid odor, and it is a noticeable odor, attracts insects for its pollination. The People taught their children "when the Skunk Cabbage is up, the ice on the lakes is no longer strong enough to walk on." Such rules are not so different from "look both ways before crossing the street."

First warning: do not eat the leaves, they cause burning in the mouth. The plant contains high levels of calcium oxalate. On occasion the root would be gathered and prepared as an infusion (tea) which was mixed with honey. The root is expectorant for asthma, bronchial problems and catarrh. It is also anti-spasmodic which helps with whooping cough. Over time other plants shared a gentler way of treating these conditions. When something as dangerous and long lasting as whooping cough came along it is understandable people tried anything that might work. If you think we have outgrown this approach, consider the process of chemotherapy and radiation. If we don't kill the person, sometimes we cure them. The way of medicine continues to improve as we learn more about plants and their way of helping. That is why I wish folks would get rid of their grass and let some medicinal plants grow in their yard.

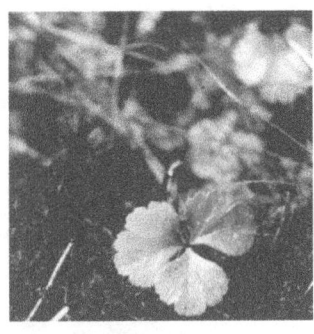

WETLANDS
Coptis groenlandica

Goldthread

There is a three leaf plant in the bog meadow. It is very small, only two inches tall, about the size of a lawn Clover. I find **Goldthread** most often growing in with the soft moss that covers fallen logs. If there is a Clover like plant growing on the log, I carefully peel the moss back to look underneath for bright yellow rootlets.

Goldthread has long root runners joining the plants of a colony and this is the part which has the medicinal gift. Gathering sections of this root requires the same kind of patience as collecting Balsam Fir sap. It is time consuming, but careful gathering keeps the plant alive and well. The moss can be replaced on the log and it will reattach. There is plenty of moisture in a bog so the plants will not dry out.

It is the yellow root, and only that part of the plant, which is needed. This little evergreen is in the Buttercup Family, which means other parts of the plant are toxic. After the roots have dried, I pour boiling water over them and let it steep for at least thirty minutes. When the liquid turns the yellow color of the root, I filter the liquid and put some in a nasal mister. This inhalant will break up the mucus in the sinuses, and works very quickly and effectively! It helps those who get sinus headaches from heavy congestion.

Goldthread has another gift as well. If someone has an infected tooth, an abscess, this root works as a poultice to draw the infection out of the jawbone. It feels strange to put little root pieces alongside a tooth, but all is forgiven when the pain stops and the swelling goes down. This is not a substitute for seeing a dentist, but it is very helpful if the infection happens when the dentist's office is closed.

Gathering in a wetland is a true test of dedication. There is no way to do it quickly, and there is the distraction of mosquitoes. I wear heavy clothes, gloves, and if needed a net hat with a face cover. I asked my grandmother why Creator made so many mosquitoes. She said it is only a problem for creatures who "have no fur! Fish and birds need the larva and the adult size mosquitoes as food." When I live outdoors in the summer the mosquitoes seem less interested in biting me. Perhaps they prefer the "exotic food" smell of a nice, fresh city person.

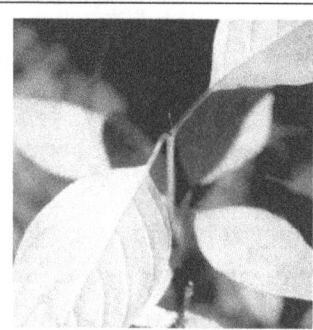

WETLANDS
Menyanthes trifoliata

Bogbean

Since your shoes are already wet we may as well look at other plants around the bog. The mossy soil is water saturated, every step squishes. Bog plants grow with their "feet in the water." There is a good sized plant growing here with three leaves at the top of a long stem. It looks like a giant Clover. If it happens to be in bloom there is a star shaped, five petal flower.

I gathered the roots of this plant for a man undergoing kidney dialysis. Only one kidney was working (somewhat) but it could not handle the toxins in his body. **Bogbean** can help the kidneys to regain balance before there is a need for dialysis. However, taking the roots means taking the life of the plant. I do not take this plant without good reason.

Bogbean is one of the plants which is now being cultivated by some of the herb supply companies. For conditions that are not immediately life threatening, I actually buy organic root from these places. This keeps the wetland meadows strong and abundant.

Bogbean is also tonic to the liver and gallbladder. These important inner organs help with digestion and overall body cleansing. Sometimes disease, over medication, or life circumstances demand more than these inner organs can manage. A plant which is tonic can be a help without being too potent.

We have already spoken about this, but lets do it again. If the digestive system is not working well it affects the entire body. Toxins escape and the lymph system must then deal with them. The spaces around the joints appear to be a prime drop zone for toxins, and it doesn't take much to interfere with a joint that needs to move freely. For chronic arthritis or rheumatism, the powdered root of Bogbean seems to help the condition. I cannot explain exactly how this works. There is no real cure for arthritis, so I don't feel lonely in my ignorance. Sometimes what matters is to work with the body to allow it to heal itself. A couple gelatin capsules of powdered Bogbean root each day could help.

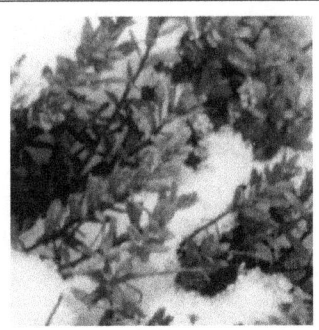

WETLANDS
Vaccinium oxycoccus

Cranberry

Remember, this is not a swamp we are looking at, this is a bog. There are strange plants growing here, most noticeable is the carpet of moss growing over the surface of the water. This is Sphagnum

Moss. I caution you not to step on the Moss, this is what might be called a quaking bog. The Moss will not support a person and you will suddenly be in water of unknown depth. However, Sphagnum Moss was an essential part of the life of the People.

The Moss clumps or sponges, are antiseptic (they contain bromine). The sponges became cloths to clean the food preparing surface, or to wash a child's face. Moss sponges were absorbent diapers for a young child, or monthly padding for a woman in her menstrual cycle. All these things benefit from the germ killing activity of the Moss, especially the young children who were free from diaper rash! For instance, Milkweed fluff would not be a good diaper because it would leak. But Sphagnum Moss will absorb ten times its own weight in water, which is a good sponge.

A bog is very acidic (but it doesn't burn your skin). There is no fresh water coming into the bog, except what falls as rain. Plants that grow near a bog are very resourceful, like the little Cranberries.

Cranberries have a slender, creeping stem up to ten inches long. The leaves are alternate, oval and pointed at the tip. The edges of the leaves are rolled under, and the leaf is white underneath. Most Cranberries are red, but I have also found white ones. The berries are easy to collect and dry. They store well, and are important in the making of winter survival food. Pemmican cakes made with fat and Cranberries, sweetened with Maple sugar, are high energy food for winter travellers.

Cranberries also have a medicinal gifting: they are a nudge to the kidneys and also help replace potassium in the body. Sometimes the ways of plants mystify me, but I am very grateful they do what they do. If someone has kidney difficulty, a Cranberry tea will help. Its native name is "Mashkigimin" which means "Medicine Berry," and it is willing to share its healing energy with people. Harvest carefully and the beds of Cranberry will be there year after year. The wild Cranberry is smaller than its domesticated relative, but it is sweeter and more reliable as a medicine.

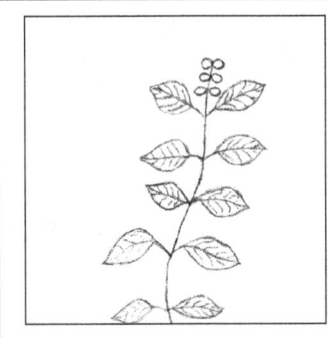

WETLANDS
Gaultheria hispidula

Creeping Snowberry

Snowberry is a trailing evergreen plant with tiny leaves. It grows in mats over mossy logs and stones. This is the same kind of place where you would find wild Cranberries, and the leaves are about the same size. I was excited when I thought I had found white Cranberries! But they were Snowberries, a cousin to the plant "Gaultheria procumbens" which is called Wintergreen.

The Snowberry has oval, dark green leathery leaves. The thick coating is to protect the plant cells from the extremes of winter. The stem is covered with stiff brown hairs, probably for the same reason.

The Indian name, "Waboozobagoons" which means "Little Snowshoe Hare Plant," is fascinating. The very young hares(they do not like being called rabbits) have a small white dot in the center of their forehead which stays there on their otherwise brown fur until they are adolescent hares. These youngsters are fun. They play tag and chase and tumble until they are too tired to move. The adults also play chase and thump their hind legs in a most interesting dance! I believe the white dot on the hare is the reason the Snowshoe Hare Plant (Snowberry) has its name. There are tiny white berries along the stem that taste very much like Wintergreen (surprise).

The People would gather the leaves for a medicinal tea. This tea is a mild stimulant and is also diaphoretic (causes sweating). It was helpful especially during the winter months for asthma or stubborn coughs. The fresh leaves could be a poultice for cuts, or wounds. A poultice is a good method for treating puncture wounds (like getting a nail in your foot). These wounds do not bleed out to cleanse themselves, so there is a high risk of infection. A winter green-leaf plant was a gift to the People. A tea that tasted good and offered the vitamins to help them through the winter was medicine that tastes good.

A swamp is sheltered from the wind, and is always warmer than the nearby woodlands. Many People had a winter wigwam in the swamp area which was frozen into dry footing until the spring thaw.

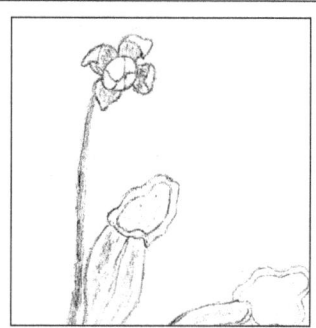

WETLANDS
Sarracenia purpurea

Pitcher Plant

There is a strange plant that grows in sphagnum bogs which my herb mother called "frog leggings." Now known as **Pitcher Plant** this odd fellow has modified leaves; leaves rounded into a smooth, hollow tube. In the tube are little hairs that all point down. Once an insect enters it becomes dinner for the plant. A bog is a low nutrient place to grow, so this clever plant uses enzymes secreted by the leaves to digest the insect and grow to be a strong, healthy plant.

The flower, which is a nodding single red bloom, is insect pollinated. Though surely some of the pollinators also wander into the pitchers. Pitcher Plant is an evergreen and the pitcher leaves can last up to two years.

This is a rare plant, and there are too few to harvest now. When the bogs were undisturbed, the People would gather the fibrous roots of this plant to make a tea for the mother to drink after the birth of a child. The leaves were sometimes used in a tea for fever and chills. Considering the two usages, I suspect the Pitcher Plant offers internal protection against infection and certain types of bacteria. One of the medicine people had a vision that this plant might be helpful for smallpox. It seemed that smallpox was nearly eradicated, and today we do not vaccinate for it. So there was no need to do further research on this plant. It is sadly ironic that one of the chemical warfare possibilities is a vigorous strain of smallpox. Perhaps it would not be such a bad idea to see to the ongoing of this plant since we do not know what the future will bring.

The plants of the swamps and bogs have very strong medicine to offer. They ask only for wetland places where they can grow in the future. I hope this will be so. I do find the insect eating plants fascinating. The two plants of this kind that I know of both choose the misty, sheltered swamps and bogs to be their home. Here they are less likely to be eaten or stepped on. Wet footing is not inviting for deer, or for clumsy humans.

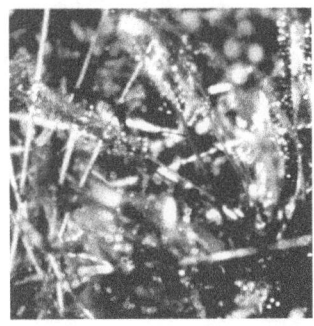

WETLANDS
Drosera species

Sundew

It would be a shame to leave the bog until you see one very beautiful little plant. The bog environment brings out the best, or at least the most unusual, in plants. It is not easy to find this plant, as its leaves are only about one fourth of an inch wide. The round leaf **Sundew** might have leaves about half an inch around, maybe.

Sunlight reflects off the moist leaf filaments of this plant making a pattern of tiny rainbows. It is called Sundew, and it is well named. This tiny plant is also carnivorous. The sticky fluid on the leaves attracts insects, then dissolves the insect after the leaf has curled around its dinner! When my herb mother first showed me this plant

I had to test it. I dropped an insect on a leaf and watched the leaf respond. Sundew has found a very clever way to get its food.

This plant is endangered, I do not gather it, but I do check every year to be sure it is still there, alive and well. I hope as we become more aware of the value of wild places, that there will be more of these special plants.

During the first World War there was little hope for soldiers who were shot in the stomach or intestinal area. These men were set aside to die, saving the bandages for those who could be helped. Two young Indian medics were horrified and asked if they could do something for these wounded. The answer was yes, but no bandages! The Indian men had noticed Sphagnum Moss growing nearby, so they gathered some and packed the wounds with it. It wasn't long before the doctors noticed the mortally wounded soldiers were not dying off, they were healing!

The little bogs are important. What if you knew that Sundew contained plumbagin which is anti-staph, strep, and pneumonia bacteria. What if you knew Sundew yields a cough syrup that can relieve the cough spasms of asthma. Perhaps if more people knew this, we could work together to protect bogs. These are important healing gifts that are no longer available to the people. I would grow a bog if I could, but I can't. So I say thank you to the mosquitoes who keep the existing bogs off the tourist maps.

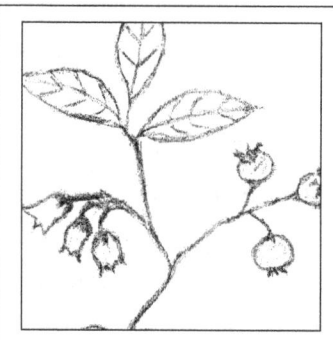

WETLANDS
Vaccinium angustifolium

Blueberries

In the long ago time when Nanabooshoo was busy travelling the land around the Great Lakes, he became hungry (this was not unusual for Nanabooshoo). The only fruits at that time were **Blueberries**, which were called "Minan, the good berries." Nanabooshoo stopped in a lowland area to pick some of the tasty blue berries. It wasn't long before he decided that stooping to harvest berries was not a proper task for "the son of the West Wind."

You must understand Nanabooshoo is a trickster figure so things don't always turn out as he expects. Nanabooshoo took a handful of berries and tossed them up on the higher ground and told them to, "be big and red, and grow on a tree" so he wouldn't have to bend over to pick them. At once apple trees came into being with lots of shiny red apples. Soon herds of deer showed up, pushed Nanabooshoo out of the way and ate all the red apples! Nanabooshoo was angry. He grabbed some half ripe apples, threw them on the ground and told them to be "fifty times bigger and right next to me so I can get them first!" Unfortunately, he didn't give any details so the crop was indeed bigger than apples…they were squash and pumpkins, but they weren't fully ripe. The caterpillars and mice ate up the crop.

Angrily Nanabooshoo grabbed some tiny green apples and threw them down on the ground. This time he didn't give any orders and up came the gourds, as bitter and inedible as the little green apples. Many times Nanabooshoo tried to get it right and other fruits came into being. Always something was not right. Finally Nanaboosho gave up saying he didn't want the fruits, he only made them for his nieces and nephews, the People. In the final scene there was Nanabooshoo back in the swamp. He was once again picking Blueberries.

The People of the Great Lakes named the North American continent "Minissa," the place where the Blueberries grow. My grandmother met two black bears when she was a tiny child. Her parents were gathering Blueberries. So were the black bears. There were berries enough for all so no harm was done except perhaps frightening her mother.

There are at least thirty species of Blueberries, they love to hybridize (genetic engineering done by the plants themselves). The different clone groups vary a little in leaf, berry shape and color.

So you will find Blueberries in dry sandy soil, in woods, along the roadside, but mostly in the wetlands. They like slightly acid soil. Blueberries grow easily in company with Oaks, Pines, and White Birch. Blueberry is somewhat shade tolerant.

Blueberries grow on a low shrub, about twelve inches tall. They grow in large patches where conditions are right. The leaves are alternate on the stems, oval and pointed. There are no thorns! There are white, bell shaped flowers, and the fruit is the Blueberry. The Blueberry flowers are insect pollinated. Just the moving wings of a bee can move the pollen from one flower to the next.

These berries are high in calcium, potassium, phosphorus and usable iron. They also contain Vitamins A, B, and C. They are tastier than Rose hips or evergreen needles for a winter vitamin supply. They dry easily (like plump, blue raisins) and they resist mold.

Blueberries not only taste good, they also have medicinal gifts to share. It is a good food for people with diabetes (diabetes is a common problem for Native American people). Blueberry is also helpful for anemia. After childbirth a Native woman would rebuild her iron supply as well as other minerals by eating Blueberries. In winter the dry berries were cooked with corn, maple sugar, wild rice, and venison. This is wonderful food.

My grandmother argued with archeologists who insisted ancient Native People did not include Blueberries in their diet. They had not found any old, dry berries at any of the sites so they wouldn't believe her. "They ate the berries, that's why you don't find them," she claimed. Finally a lone, very dry Blueberry was found at an archeological dig, and my grandmother was delighted.

Who else eats Blueberries? Almost all birds who can balance on the branches. Also chipmunks, skunks, white-footed mice (they look like they have socks on), and of course, black bears. People still eat Blueberries because they are tasty, and so do bears. Leave enough for other beings when you go to pick the berries, it is part of the balance of all life.

Water & Shoreline

Most of the oxygen in our air is the gift of aquatic plants (especially the much maligned algae). These plants must continue for the life of any air breathing creature on this planet.

This is a very different world for plants, this water world, and the plants have found marvellous ways of adapting to it. Some grow near shore where their roots can find a solid base while the leaves reach up into the air to capture sunlight. Others have floating leaves with waxy coatings and tiny air holes for breathing. Some have floating leaves and no roots at all; they go wherever the wind or the gentle current takes them. The deep water plants have roots holding firmly to the bottom while their leaves absorb the sunlight that filters down to them through the water. Wherever the plants live, they offer shelter and food to the other creatures of the water.

To experience these plants you need a boat, or you can go wading. During one of my first lessons in plants I followed my herb mother out into a swamp. She was not collecting plants, she was offering Kinnik and greeting these plants in the early summer.

White sneakers take on a dark grey color from water adventures and are ever after called expendable swamp shoes.

In the shallow water of a lake are the emergent plants. They are adapted to changing water levels and have wide spreading roots. These roots hold the sediment and slow the force of the incoming waves. They have creative reproductive methods. When the water level is low they produce seeds. When the water level is high they produce new plants from their roots, or rhizomes.

Out beyond the emergents are the floating leaf plants. A colony of water lilies holds the sediment in the deeper places. The leaf stems grow quickly and the rounded leaves float easily on the surface. The flowers are above the water so that insect pollinators can reach them and still stay dry.

From shoreline to deep water the plants form a balanced community. They are there for fish, frog, turtle, muskrat and even long legged wading birds. All are welcome and share in the bounty of these plants.

WATER & SHORELINE
Calla palustris

Water Arum

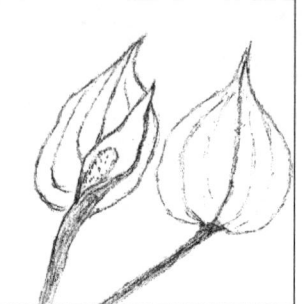

WATER & SHORELINE
Peltandra virginica

Arrow Arum

Water Arum is a beautiful plant growing maybe seven inches tall in the shallow waters of a marsh or bog. The leaves are wide and heart shaped growing on a long thick stalk (in case the water rises). The root is a fleshy rhizome with many tiny rootlets to hold it in place. The flower is magnificent. A white flower leaf forms a funnel shaped cloak around a spike of tiny flowers. The shape helps the insects and pond snails to pollinate the plants more efficiently. The red berries form on a flower stalk and can drop easily into the water for future Water Arum. It is amazing how plants of a place adapt to the creatures who can help them continue their cycle of reproduction.

Water Arum loves shallow peat bogs and mucky sediment of quiet ponds. It grows in linked colonies or solitary clumps which grow from rhizomes or seeds. Water Arum is a good food plant for wetland birds who gladly leave the "processed" berries in the pond for the future. Muskrats eat the roots and leaves. A fleshy rhizome is also a possible food source for people since it can be dried and pounded into flour for bread. Since there are many places where corn and wheat will not grow, here other plants offer a substitute for survival.

The **Arrow Arum** also likes the shallow water. It sends "arrow" shaped leaves up above the water to a height of twelve inches or more.

The flower has a green cloak to shelter the white-orange flower spadix. The roots are thick and fibrous, and they spread to provide solid footing for the plant. The seeds form clusters of greenish berries which have a gelatinous coating. They are less inviting to bird consumers but can float safely in the water to find a suitable place to grow.

The Indian name for Arrow Arum is "Tikibughoose," which means "Leaf That Cools." It suggests perhaps the leaves were used to lower a fever. In the bog areas there are not the familiar plants like Catnip which will lower a fever. The Medicine People sometimes dreamed of plants living in the wet places, praying that they share their gifts with the People. Plants have not stopped talking to people, it is more that people no longer listen to the Plants.

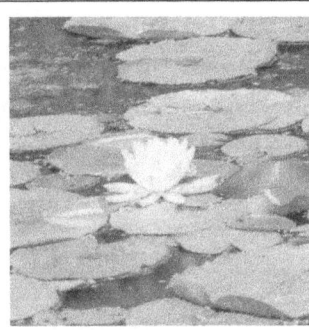

WATER & SHORELINE
Nymphaea odorata

White Water Lily

Where the water is calm in a pond or near the shore of a lake, you find the **Water Lilies**. Out from the shore in water about four feet deep, the Lily pads float on the surface. They are attached to the bottom of the lake by long thick stems, with four air passages that bring oxygen to the under-water parts of the plant. The thick leathery green leaves are purplish underneath, but the green topsides show chlorophyll is working with the energy of the sun to feed the plant. This is a perennial water plant and the food for winter and spring is stored in the interconnected system of root/rhizomes.

White Water Lilies are now legally protected, but before the lakes were disturbed by boats and jet skis, there were many White Lilies with their edible roots. Why would an Indian go digging around in pond muck looking for dinner? I don't think it happened that way. Sometimes the tubers lose their grip on the bottom and float to the surface. Someone in a canoe might reach down for the potato-like rhizome and find it tasted pretty good. It tasted even better roasted! There are also seeds in the beautiful white flowers. Imagine their surprise when someone roasted the seeds to save for winter and found the seeds popped, just like popcorn!

The seeds are not only for humans, the water birds also know what is good to eat. It is a good thing there are many rhizomes, as they also feed porcupine, muskrat, beaver, deer and moose. Deer and moose know the leaves and flowers are tasty as greens, so it did not take long for the People to learn this as well.

The People also learned this White Lily was a strong medicine plant, believed to belong to the underwater Spirits. The floating leaves are styptic and make a good poultice for bleeding wounds. A tea or infusion made from the tuber help with all kinds of breathing difficulties. For swollen glands, cough and symptoms of tuberculosis, this was the plant they asked for help. Some of the dried rhizomes were kept for winter food, but equally as many were stored for the gift of healing.

The People understand their relationship to the waters, from small ponds to the Great Lakes. A canoe is a very fragile craft in waters with swift current, or when the shore is out of sight. Offerings were placed to show respect to the Spirits of these places. Remember, the Lake thinks nothing of sinking a huge freighter even in our time!

WATER & SHORELINE
Nuphar variegata

Yellow Pond Lily

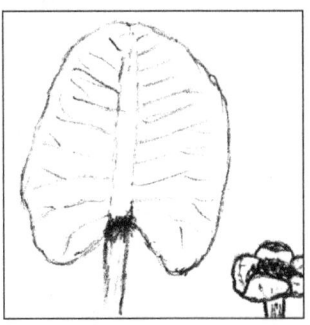

WATER & SHORELINE
Nelumbo lutea

American Lotus

Yellow Pond Lily is more common in still water places. It has oval leathery floating leaves with lobes that overlap at the stem. Its yellow flowers blossom all summer long, standing several inches above the surface of the water. This water lily is not protected, so if you want to make a popcorn-like snack, use the seeds of this plant (after giving an offering, of course). The tuber roots are large and fleshy and will cook like a potato.

The **American Lotus** is a fascinating plant, as well. It is related to the Asian Lotus which is classified as *Nelumbo nucifera*. The Lotus chooses water a little shallower than the Water Lilies, maybe two feet deep. The plant structure is also somewhat different. The leaves are a blue-green color, and some of these leaves are above the water surface. The supporting stem attaches in the center of the lower side of the leaf. Viewed from the side this gives the leaf a funnel-like appearance.

The flower is a misty yellow color. The seed pod is a spongy greenish-yellow pod with seeds on its surface. When the seed container dries it breaks loose from the stem and floats away upside down scattering seeds as it goes. Some of these seeds can stay dormant for hundreds of years, a powerful way of seeing to the future.

At one time, when these plants were more abundant, the People ground the dry seeds to make a sweet tasting meal (somewhat like oatmeal) with a high energy content. They gathered the banana shaped tubers and roasted them like potatoes. If there were extra tubers the women would slice the tubers length wise and hang the pieces to dry in the rafters of the wigwam for winter food.

The growing season of the northern Great Lakes is short, and not well suited to domestic gardening. The People learned from the plants of the place which ones had food energy enough to share. In fall the People gathered these plants and saved them for the six months of winter soon to come.

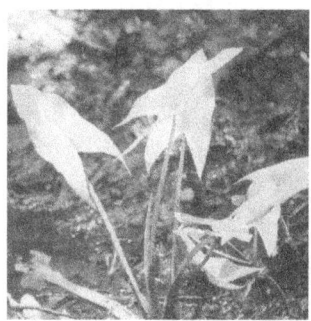

WATER & SHORELINE
Sagittaria latifolia

Arrowroot

A healthy wetland will feed a lot of shoreline birds. Where **Arrowroot** grows you may well see ducks with their tails in the air dabbling in the bottom for the tasty little white corms that form among the mass of roots. These pinkish-white little bulbs also feed muskrats, beavers and people. The corms are about two inches long and one inch wide. They are somewhat sweet and starchy. The People of the Great Lakes called the Arrowroot "Wabasi Pin" which means "White Potato." They would boil the corms like potatoes, slice them, then hang them from the rafters of the wigwam to dry. They looked almost like Christmas trim on their strings. The dry slices could then become a part of a stew or soup at any time of the year.

There was nearly always a fire in the wigwams of the people, or outside the lodge during the warm days of summer. A soup was kept warm at the fire to feed the family or to feed those who came to visit.

It was an obligation to offer food where the rigors of winter or travel made food a matter of life or death. A traveller could expect food from anyone who was of the same clan, as these were "relatives" even if they came from another village.

The corms are a method of reproduction for the Arrowroot, sprouting into large colonies. The leaves are arrow shaped and grow in water from three inches to three feet deep. The flowers grow from their own stalk. The male flowers have three white petals, and above them on the stalk are rounded balls which are the female flowers. These balls have many tiny nutlets waiting for pollination by a passing insect.

The leaves of the Arrowroot have been used as medicine for rheumatism. The tubers were made into a tea for indigestion. It is not surprising these two conditions meet in the same plant. There is often a connection between improper digestion and certain forms of arthritis.

Sometimes the muskrats would harvest more corms than they could eat and would bury the excess in little caches. Finding such a cache a woman might offer Kinnik and take some of the corms to feed her family. It was part of the balance for her to leave enough corms for the Muskrat family also.

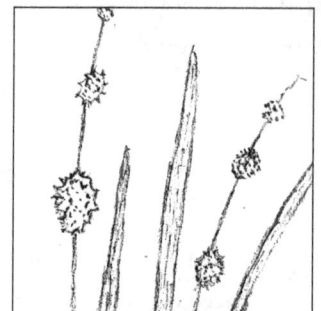

WATER & SHORELINE
Sparganium species

Bur Reed

WATER & SHORELINE
Scirpus validus

Bulrush

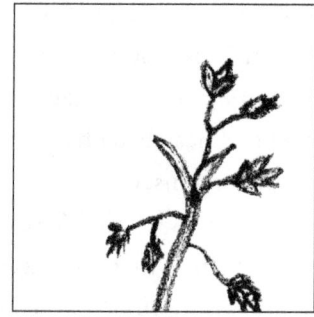

Sometimes its not all about us, the humans that is. I think Creator made this plant especially for waterfowl and shoreline birds. **Bur Reed** grows to four feet above the water surface. The stems are a sturdy triangular shape, and make an interesting sound when the wind blows them against each other. The leaves are long and narrow like cattail leaves, but it also has both floating and submerged leaves.

The rhizomes spread out and build colonies of these Bur Reed plants (many species). For genetic strength and variability, Bur Reed also produces flowers. The flower stalk grows up in a zig-zag pattern. The blossoms are spaced along these stalks like little fishing weights. The Bur Reed makes the upper blossoms male, about half an inch in size. The lower female flowers are twice the size. The male and female flowers of a single plant mature at different times so there is always cross pollination from another mature plant whose flowering cycle matches up. The wind blows among the reeds making music and fertilizing the flowers. The little fuzzy flower balls then dry and become prickly like burrs. These fruits are a feast for mallard ducks and swans. The varying heights of the Bur Reed makes it a wonderful nesting site for many water birds.

The young birds in the nursery can listen to the dance sound of their safe little nursery.

Bulrush has a long sturdy rounded stem that can grow to seven feet tall. Bulrush likes water about three feet deep where the bottom is firm. This rush also offers good nesting sites for waterfowl. The tall rushes make the nest almost invisible to predators.

People have also favored the tall strong reeds. Their stems are the same thickness all the way up, and there are no joints in their stems. The ivory colored dry rushes could be woven into watertight baskets. The pale rushes could also be dyed to offer a weaver a choice of colors for her baskets. Some of these baskets are very beautiful. Funny, we offer weaving mainly to our elders as a recreation in an old age home, when the dexterity of young fingers could weave more easily, and weaving is enjoyable.

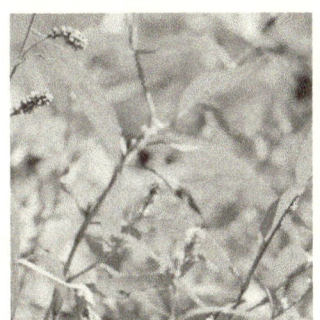

WATER & SHORELINE
Polygonum amphibium

Water Smartweed

WATER & SHORELINE
Chelone glabra

Turtlehead

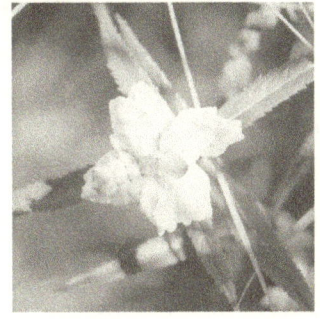

Water Smartweed is a very adaptable plant. It can be one to five feet tall, and can grow on land or in shallow water where it produces floating leaves. This plant has long narrow leaves and tiny pink flowers on slender spikes about an inch long. The flowers look like the Smartweed has sprouted birthday candles. The abundant seeds are good food for ducks and geese. These birds look for such plants to feed them along their migration routes.

The People gathered some of the leaves for medicine. A poultice of fresh leaves would clean and help heal skin ulcers. A tea made from dried leaves helped with stomach ache, as Water Smartweed has a mild pain reliever action. This infusion also releases "rutin" which strengthens tiny capillary walls to prevent internal bleeding. Perhaps the Native gatherers did not use these words to describe the medicine, but they were aware that certain conditions were improved by the gift of this plant.

Turtlehead has a good common name, because the pinkish white flower with its swollen upper lip resembles a turtle's head. Turtlehead grows about two feet tall with lance shaped opposite leaves. The stem is somewhat square, but most apparent are the flower clusters at the top of the plant.

An ointment made from fresh ground leaves was used for inflamed breasts in a nursing mother. This condition needs help, or the feeding of a newborn is very painful. True, there are bottles for feeding now, but that milk does not share the immunities of a mother with her child. Also, there is rarely an allergic reaction to mother's milk, in fact it seems well designed to feed newborn human children.

This same Turtlehead ointment is also good medicine for skin ulcers and cold sores. There is a cleansing activity suited to tender skin which is, perhaps, the kindest gift of this plant. I am somewhat concerned that our medical researchers do not look for medicine well suited to the condition. Some of our medicines appear too general, or do more harm than good. Plants have always been willing to share their healing gifts if we ask in a good way. For many reasons we need the Plants to survive.

WATER & SHORELINE
Pontedaria cordata

Pickerelweed

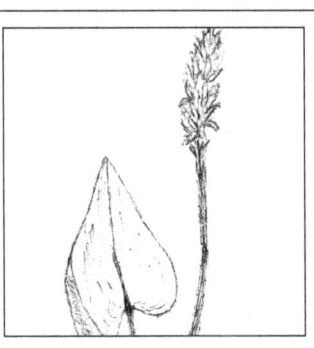

WATER & SHORELINE
Alisma plantago-aquatica

Water Plantain

There is a city in Wisconsin near Lake Michigan called Kenosha, and its name means Pickerel, after a dark green fish with stripes on its body. The People called this plant "Kinozhaegunzh," which means "Pickerel Plant." **Pickerelweed** has many fine parallel veins (stripes) along its glossy, heart shaped leaves. The stems are tall and strong, they allow air to move down to the roots for food making.

Blue flowers with tiny yellow dots form along a long spike. The lowest flowers bloom first, followed by the upper flowers througout the summer. Each individual flower lasts for only one day. These little flowers are very rich in nectar and attract bees to help with pollination. Like many other water plants, Pickerelweed also has rhizomes which spread into colonies.

The flower stalks are great resting places for flying insects. The seeds are food for wetland birds and animals. Also important, the leaves and stems make shady, protected places for fish to hide. Pickerelweed is sturdy enough to break wave trains and shelter other water plants from rough water currents.

Water Plantain prefers the shallow water, or even wet mud. Like the land Plantain, Water Plantain leaves grow in a basal rosette and have prominent parallel veins. The root tubers help spread the plant, as do the seeds that form in a little tightly packed ring from many tiny flowers.

Songbirds like to perch on the old stems, and the tubers and seeds feed the ducks. Beavers eat the leaves and the tubers. I suppose that is why so many of these plants have both seeds and rhizomes; so many creatures depend on them for food.

Raw Water Plantain leaves can irritate the skin. It is the root which offers the medicinal gifting to people. An infusion of rhizome is diuretic and a tonic to the liver. It helps prevent fatty deposits which interfere with liver function. This same infusion also helps lower blood pressure and glucose levels. It is good for diabetics. Many Native Americans are prone to diabetes, so this was a welcome medicine plant. Water Plantain root infusion also helps prevent kidney stone formation and urinary tract problems. This plant has many gifts. We need more clean wetlands to grow such good plants.

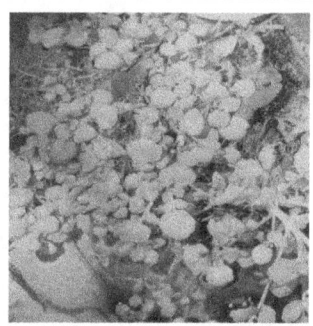

WATER & SHORELINE
Nasturtium officinale

Watercress

Watercress is a perennial which grows in colonies during all four seasons of the year. It likes clear moving water where it can reach up to two feet tall. The leaves are divided into leaflets, as many as nine leaflets or as few as three. Watercress is in the Mustard family, and the leaves are tasty raw or cooked. The leaves contain Vitamins C, E, A, and also Iodine.

A river with a strong current does not always freeze over in winter. Where the People found drinking water in the winter, they also found fresh greens for vitamins and minerals. Even dry Watercress leaves offer help for vitamin deficiency, so these were gathered and dried for the coldest months. The Vitamin E also helped with stamina and endurance. The People used fresh Watercress as a tonic, a delicious way to get the blood moving at the end of winter. Winter meant a lot of time spent indoors and the body welcomed the energy boost to prepare for Spring.

There are still many places where Watercress grows in abundance, but we must be certain the river is clean. The plants have no choice but to live where they are born. We need to be aware of what might be a pollution source for a body of water. This is true for all of the water plants as well as the land plants. I hope we will soon realize what a danger pollution is to ourselves and our children. Pollution does not have to be there, but somehow we put it there in our haste for profit in industry. There are too many environmentally caused diseases for us to ignore this problem. Rivers clean themselves quickly, as their water bubbles over gravel beds letting the air do the cleansing work.

Watercress makes a nice salad green and still offers its gift of purifying the blood. This means less opportunity for rheumatism as well as help for the kidneys and liver. Wouldn't it be nice if our food were also medicine? It is! Plants that grow here by their own choice have far more food value to offer than processed foods. Someone once said, "if your food has a list of ingredients, it's not food."

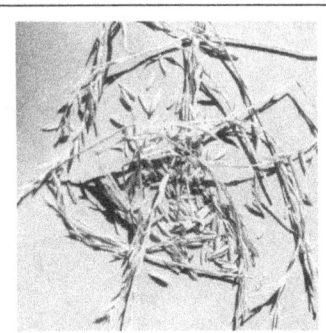

WATER & SHORELINE
Zizania palustris

Wild Rice

Long ago, when the People of the Great Lakes came to the Eastern shores of North America, they became concerned they would lose their tribal identity by living with the People on the coast. Their homeland had been destroyed and they were grateful to have survived, but the elders were concerned. A number of elders went off to fast and pray about the situation. One of the elders had a vision:

> A great Megis (cowrie) shell rose out of the water and offered to lead the People to the Place which would be their homeland. They would not have to fight a war to live in this Place. The Shell told the elder the Place would have great seas of fresh water. Most important, there would be "food growing on the water." After a long, long time following the Spirit Megis they came to the inland seas. Here, indeed, was food growing on the water, Mahnomin, Wild Rice.

Wild Rice likes shallow water. The places where the Rice grows thickest are harvested by the families of that area. They come early enough to honor the Rice before the harvest begins. When the Rice is ripe there is a ceremonial harvest first. Two women and one man collect enough for a feast. The Wild Rice kernels are tapped off the plant into the bottom of the canoe. While the feast is prepared the men sing songs to honor the Rice.

After the harvest the Wild Rice dries slowly in the sun. When dry it is baked for about three hours over a low fire. Then the Rice is threshed by pounding it with sticks, then walking on it with new moccasins. It is winnowed by pouring the Rice from tray to tray letting the chaff be blown away by the wind. The Wild Rice is then ready to cook, or to be stored for other days.

Wild Rice is good nutritious food. It cooks longer than other rices, needing about an hour. It needs extra water too, as it swells a lot, about six cups of water to one cup of Wild Rice. It is very, very good. Wild Rice was and still is a staple for the People. The growing season is too short for most potatoes, but the Wild Rice does well, and the harvesters make sure enough seed is left to insure the Rice will continue. The Plants share all we need to be strong and healthy. Surely we can see to it that they can continue their life cycle here, for themselves and for all living creatures.

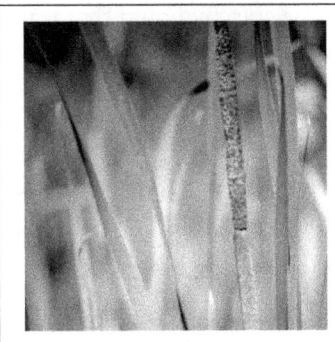

WATER & SHORELINE
Typha latifolia

Cattail

In the shallow water there is a large colony of **Cattails**, some have wider leaves (*latifolia*, about one inch wide), some have slender leaves (*angustafolia*, about one half inch wide). You may notice some are halfway between the two sizes, but don't talk about those, as scientists say that they don't exist!

My herb mother called Cattails the defenders of the shoreline. These tall ones hold their place, and settle the water currents that might wash away plants with lesser root structures.

With Cattail it seems its physical being is also its spiritual gifting, as it is food and shelter to many animals. The male and female flowers are on the same plant, but the flowers are modified into bristles which hold large amounts of pollen. Wind does the pollinating, but Cattails take no chances. If the pollen fails they can spread through their rootstock.

In early spring we could gather some of the young shoots to eat like asparagus. The muskrats also think this is good food. We could wait a little longer and gather some of the new green flower spikes and boil them in our soup. Other times I try not to interfere with pollination except to gather a little of the golden pollen that forms on the Cattail heads.

To do this I take a brown paper bag, put it over the Cattail, and gently shake some of the pollen into the bag. Then I release the Cattail to continue its reproductive journey. The pollen looks almost like corn meal, and mixed with flour it makes high energy pancakes.

There are also salad crunchies growing at the bottom of the stalks, right above where the stem meets the root. The stalk base is a crispy, white edible that tastes great in a salad. The starchy liquid that leaks out of the stem will work to thicken a soup, so no flour is needed to make stew.

The People lived on the hilltops in summer to avoid the mosquitoes, and Cattail helped with this as well. The long Cattail leaves were sewn together at the base to form door and window coverings to let in air but to keep out insects. The mature Cattail heads are also marvellous insulation material for mittens, blankets and clothing. Yes, it needs to be quilted to keep it from bunching, but then so does goosedown. Cattail down is easier on the geese.

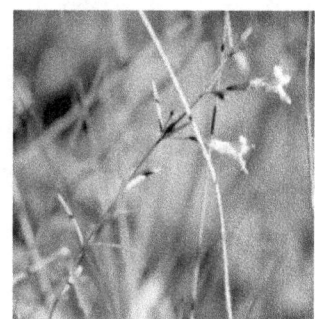

WATER & SHORELINE
Satureja arkansa

Calamint

We walk now along the shore of the Great Lake. This place is very different, the Earth itself vibrates in response to the rhythm of the waves breaking on the shore. There is a loud drumbeat as the waves drop onto the rocks, then there is a rattling of smaller stones as the water runs back again to the Lake.

We look to the swale to find this little Mint. The swale is the lower ground near the shore, behind the mound of rock and sand pushed up onto the shore by the waves. The swale is wet from water that comes in during storms, or when the time of high water lets some waves flow over the shoreline mound. The Great Lakes have a pattern of tides, but we are supposed to call it a seiche since this is not the ocean.

When the hero, Nanabooshoo, was doing a journey around the Great Lakes, he encountered the Spirit of the Lake which is the Great Sturgeon, Nahma. Nanabooshoo always worried the People, since some of his doings didn't turn out so well. The People asked Nanabooshoo to catch the Great Sturgeon. Actually, they hoped the Sturgeon would swallow Nanabooshoo, which it did!

Nanabooshoo was able to escape the Sturgeon by chopping his way out. The People were horrified, there could be no relationship with the waters of the Great Lakes without the Spirit of the Lake. So Nanabooshoo hurried to put the Great Sturgeon back together with the help of his father, the West Wind. The Sturgeon came back to life but some of the blood of the Great Fish was left on the beach. It was absorbed by a tiny plant growing along the shore. This plant is called "Nahmahbinigunzh," which means Plant of the Sturgeon. When it begins its growth cycle the stem is green. But when the blooms appear the stem turns red to remind the People of the gift of the Sturgeon.

Nahmahbinigunzh is a small perennial mint which grows four to eight inches tall. The leaves are oval at the base of the plant, the upper leaves are long and narrow. The plant has a strong Pennyroyal scent to it.

A tea made with the above ground part of the plant is a relaxant. It is not a sedative that will make you sleep, instead it calms jangley nerves to let you sleep. The way of our society sometimes makes it difficult for people to let go of the events of the day, so it is a healing gift of Nahmahbinigunzh to help with this problem. A cup of tea, one teaspoon dry plant to a cup of boiling water, helps the body relax.

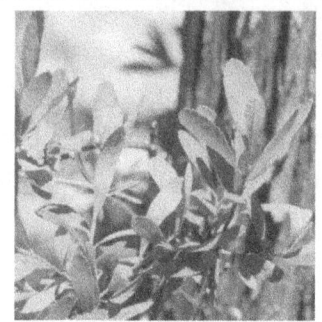

WATER & SHORELINE
Myrica gale

Sweet Gale

This is a fragrant shrub that grows in the swales near the shores of the Great Lakes. It shares these wet places with Shrub Willow, so where you find Willow you may also find Sweet Gale. Most of the Sweet Gale plants in a colony are about four feet tall. The male flowers grow on one plant, the female flowers on another. Interestingly, the shrubs alternate this sexual identity. One year a given bush may be male, another year it may be female. It may be that the minerals needed to determine sexual identity may be more abundant in one place or another (adaptable plant!).

The Sweet Gale grows with its "feet in the water." The shrubs have many branches and little hairy branchlets. The leaves are a gray-green color and stand upright on their stems. Each oval leaf tip has notches at the tip that look like little teeth standing upright.

The other noticeable features are the tiny glands under the leaves. This plant is related to Bayberry with a fragrance that comes from the tiny leaf glands. The People did not prepare any internal medicines from this plant. Rather Sweet Gale was asked to share its sweet fragrant leaves as one of the plants in Kinnikinnik. This mixture of dry plants is a part of the prayers and also a way to say thank you to other beings. When I gather plants, I place a small offering of Kinnik at the ground near the plant I wish to gather. I say "thank you" and tell the plant how it will be used for the People. There is also an obligation to see to the ongoing of these plants, so I do not overharvest, and I make sure the place is reseeded for the future.

Sweet Gale is a legume. The roots have a relationship with nitrogen fixing bacteria. This allows for a deep, rich green leaf color, and also helps to build a richer soil where the water meets the shoreline. The action of the waves brings in some nutrients, but it also removes nutrients from the soil. Sweet Gale and other plants alter their environment in fascinating ways. Many times they build up the soil so that other plants can come after them and find what they need to live. I wish we humans could learn this kind of relationship with the Earth. There is enough for all if we can find a proper balance with other forms of life.

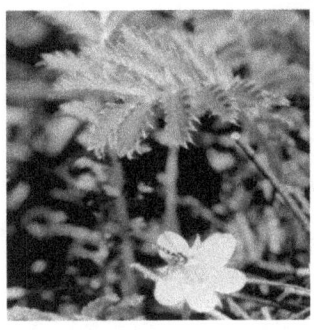

WATER & SHORELINE
Potentilla anserina

Silverweed

Along the beach, among the stones and the sturdy grasses and shoreline reeds, we find *Potentilla*. It is a beautiful plant with a golden yellow flower to mark its time of blooming. This plant grows in colonies attached by above ground fuzzy red runners. The leaves alternate on the stem and have serrated edges. It is the underside of these leaves that gives rise to its common name, **Silverweed**. The underneath of the leaves is a silvery gray color.

A well filtered infusion of leaves was used as an eyewash by the People. The leaves themselves, freshly picked, were placed inside the moccasins as a liner to give rest to tired feet. Something in the leaves is medicinal and healing to the small bones and tendons of the foot.

My herb mother gathered many fresh *Potentilla* leaves, pounded and ground them with a smooth rock into a wet pulp. She then soaked this overnight in glycerin and some other fragrant things that allowed the inner essence of the plant to drain into the liquid. This liquid was then mixed into a cream base to make a massage liniment. The liniment is good for tired feet and tired hands. I have given it to people who show symptoms of carpal tunnel syndrome. It seems to help with the internal swelling that comes from repetitive motion.

The way of medicinal plants is time consuming, but I can't think of a better way to spend time. When I view Plants as People, each walk is a chance to be with a friend. These friends let me share their home and teach me about life as they see it. Plants and rocks have a different view of time. They think we humans are hyperactive, as we never stay in one place long enough to see what is really there, or to understand what is really important.

Where land and water come together is a special place. I watch little water snakes go out and catch a minnow dinner. They rest silently in the water like stems of plants, until a willing fish comes near. After dinner the snake takes a rest in the warm sand. It doesn't take much to keep a snake happy. Perhaps it is the same for us. The People called this the Great Mystery, the Plan of the Creator for all Life on Earth. Our purpose as the People is to learn about this Plan and go along with it…simple, eh?

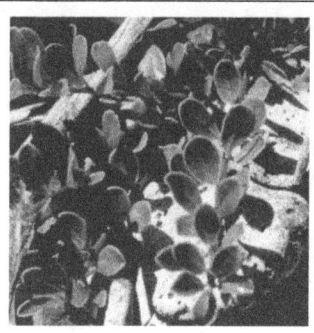

WATER & SHORELINE
Arctostaphylos uvaursi

Bearberry

Bearberry leaves look the same in spring, summer and fall. They even look much the same under a covering of snow. This is a short plant, always flat on the ground, with oval glossy leaves. The leaves are quite stiff and almost look waxed (which they are, in a plant-kind of fashion.) The blossoms are lantern shaped (like Blueberries), white with a pink border. Bearberry loves to grow on calcareous limestone beaches which is the terrain of the northern Great Lakes.

I gather a lot of Bearberry every summer. It requires care and consideration, as this is a slow growing plant. The leaf stems come off a woody runner that takes many years to grow and spread. I cut a few new growth runners from the Bearberry patches along the beach. If you find Bearberry, please don't pull it, as that will destroy many years of growth.

Bearberry leaves are antiseptic and astringent to the urogenital systems of the body. They are antilithic (stones) and anti-microbial. It is a wonder that this plant can stop internal bleeding. Bearberry is tonic to the kidneys, and very helpful to people who are borderline diabetics. Bearberry is a diuretic, and is wonderful for healing bladder infections, especially in combination with Yarrow. Even more fascinating, a strong Bearberry infusion helps shrink fibroid cysts.

Bearberry tea tastes pretty good, and I make it like sun tea. I put two handfuls of dry leaves (about half a cup) into a gallon glass jar. I pour a gallon of boiling water over the leaves and screw on the lid. It can steep a long time because of the thick coating on the leaves. The tea is ready when the leaves sink to the bottom of the jar, then filter and drink. My grandmother drank this tea every day, and she lived to be eighty-six, a long life for a Native American diabetic. Any plant called by the name of Bear is very strong medicine.

Like Cedar, the Bearberry leaves take a long time to dry. I spread them inside brown paper bags, as they turn brown if they get too much sunlight while drying. I save the Bearberry leaves from making tea, dry them again, then put them into my Kinnik mixture. This is the only commandment of the People: Do Not Waste. Perhaps saving the Bearberry leaves for prayers is also my way to remember the physical and the spiritual aspects of things do not come apart.

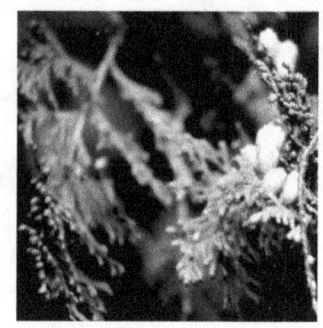

WATER & SHORELINE
Thuja occidentalis

White Cedar

"Nokomis Giizhick," the **White Cedar**, is the Tree of Life for the People. It is one of two trees which made it possible for the People to survive in the place of the Great Lakes. Its leaves are tiny and pale green, and look like overlapping scales. Their strong fragrance comes from tiny oil glands underneath the leaves. The leaves grow in fan-like sprays that catch the sun, whether the tree is growing in the swamp or along the shore of the Lakes. The cones are plump, green and oily early in the summer season. They turn a woody brown at the end of the season. Cedar bark is brown, thin and fibrous. So you know cedar boxes are not made from Cedar, but from Juniper trees.

Cedar is wind pollinated, but can also grow from the trunk of a fallen tree, a nurse tree. Often you will see the line of Cedars growing from an old log, part of the Symbolism of the Tree of Life, always renewing itself.

Grandmother Cedar has a story that will help you understand how she came to the People:

> Long ago, at the time of Creation, the Animal Beings of this Planet were told to watch over each other, that whatever happened to one affected all the others. After a while the creatures below the Earth and the creatures above the Earth lost touch with each other.
>
> One of the "on the Earth" species began to sicken. The birds, the creatures of the "above the Earth," noticed first because they have the best perspective. The birds didn't know what to do and wanted to ask the "below ground" creatures for help. They wanted Beaver to take a message down for

them since he could travel under the ground, but Beaver was "too busy." Beaver finally decided to help when a persistent Eagle swooped down and parted his fur a couple times. The "below ground" animals then called a council to talk about the problem of the sickly animal. Bear and Otter spoke in favor of helping the sick animals, so they were made a committee to do something about the problem.

Bear wanted to dig an opening up from the great underground den to communicate with other creatures, but none of the trees that Beaver brought to do the job were good for digging. Some were brittle, some were sticky, some were too heavy! Finally Bear asked Creator for a tree that was light weight, slippery, flexible and wouldn't rot when it got wet. Creator gave Bear the Cedar Tree, and that worked very well.

The sickly humans were pounding bark (for baskets) near the Lake. When the adult humans saw Bear coming they ran away. They were so frightened they forgot one of their babies who was crying loudly. Bear didn't think he could speak that "crying language," but when he looked into the child's mouth he saw what was the matter. The baby didn't have a" last berry" to keep the others down, the one that dangles at the back of the throat.

Bear slid down a slope and a new plant began to grow, a plant called Bearberry. Bear put the red berry in the child's mouth and the crying stopped. He also promised to help the People with other medicines as well. When Bear replanted the Cedar there was a new tree which lived on all three levels, below, on, and above the Earth. This was the "Tree that saved the People," the White Cedar.

One of the gifts of Cedar is the oil from the new cones. Cedar oil is a part of all of the Life Ceremonies of the People, from birth to passing over. The Cedar boughs make a waterproof covering for a shelter. Dry Cedar boughs can be burned and used as a fumigant because the smoke is antiseptic. The outer bark can be used to weave containers and floor mats that repel moths and prevent mold. The wood does not rot in water, and was used as frame wood for canoes.

When the colonists came to America many were suffering from rickets, there were no Vitamin C tablets at that time. Cedar tea was a tasty and available evergreen, and the tea worked to prevent rickets! However, steep Cedar tea for only one minute, so that it does not leach out the tannins which people do not need. Mild Cedar tea will settle your stomach and is also a breath freshener.

Cedar is one of two plants that must be a part of Kinnikinnik. The other plant is Bearberry. There are many fragrant plants that are also welcome in the mixture. "Kinnik" means "Mixed," and saying the word twice means "much mixed." Kinnikinnik is the tobacco which is part of the prayers of the People of the Great Lakes area (called Chippewa by the government).

Please remember that the word "Nokomis," which is part of the name for Cedar, is the word for "Grandmother." Nokomis is a proper title whether the elder is your relative, or an elder who has earned a title of respect.

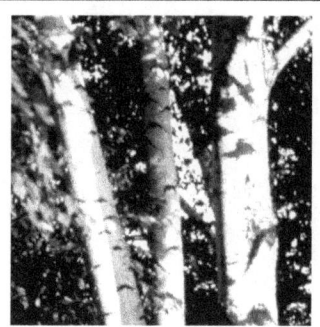

WATER & SHORELINE
Betula papyrifera

White Birch

As surely as there is a Grandmother tree, so is there a Grandfather tree. As it is said in the prayers, "May there always be balance." This is "Mishomis Wigwaas," Grandfather Birch. Birch has a tall, shimmery white trunk with chevrons; black markings along the bark that look like Thunderbirds!

This is the tree to find if there is a sudden thunderstorm, as a Birch will not be struck by lightning. A story says this was a gift from the Thunderbirds who brought lightning to the Earth. Scientists should probably analyze the sap of this tree to figure out why this is so.

Whichever way you view things, this is the other tree that made it possible for the People to survive here in the Place where the "food grows on the water" (Wild Rice). Our society has worked very hard to separate clear scientific reasoning from the murky depths of legend and mythology. I walk the woods with one foot in each world.

The People of the Great Lakes wandered from place to place following the patterns of the seasons, and their curiosity about the Land given to them by Creator. Lakes and rivers were the pathways for their beautiful Birchbark canoes. On the Great Lakes "great canoes" were paddled by ten or twelve men. Almost everything that was needed for life was made from Birch or Cedar. A Birchbark canoe is very beautiful. The Cedar frame is light weight, water resistant, and flexible enough to bend into shape. Long sheets of Birchbark are sewn (or lashed) into place to cover the frame of the canoe.

The Birchbark strips are cut on a certain day in late winter. If it is done properly, at the right time, and with cuts the proper depth, the bark pops off the tree without damaging the cambium layer of the Birch tree. This was one of the skills which was carefully taught and handed down generation to generation by the People.

Birchbark provided a lightweight flexible material to make their household complete. For cooking and water storage there were Birchbark "makuks." They looked like pails, but were wide at the bottom and narrow at the top. Birchbark is waterproof, so they only needed some Pine pitch along the seams to be water tight. The lids for the storage makuks were also water tight, so food could be stored for winter use. The plates, bowls, and cups were also Birch; easy to make and light weight. Pottery dishes just weren't practical for woodland people who walked, or canoed from place to place.

The wigwams (not tepees, those are west of the Mississippi River) were also made of Birchbark. They are domed shelters perfect for summer or winter living. The People bent long Cornus boughs, which are very flexible, to form a frame then covered it with long strips of Birchbark. In winter they added an inner layer of woven Cedar mats, then filled the space between the walls with Cattail fluff insulation. There was a central firepit and an adjustable smoke hole in the roof.

The People used tightly rolled strips of Birchbark for torches. They wound the strips around the end of a heavy pole so light could travel with them at night. Out in canoes after dark, the light of the torches attracted fish for spearing. Birchbark is very effective for firemaking, it is highly flammable. You can take a thin strip of bark, soak it in water, shake the water off, and it will light like dry paper! I tell you that in case you wondered how the People got a fire going in the rain.

The inner bark of Birch can be cooked as a survival soup. This is not a delicious broth, but there is enough nutrition in it to keep you alive. The inner bark, the cambium layer of a tree, is the layer where the life sap moves from the roots to the leaves. In the spring of the year the Birch trees run sap as the Maples do. It can be evaporated down as syrup or sugar, though it is slightly less sweet.

Birch likes the cool temperatures of the boreal forests. They are wind pollinated, forming catkins early in the spring. Birch is also somewhat fire dependent, and grows very well from burned over stumps. In doing away with small seasonal forest fires, we have not done well for the many plants and trees who need this in their life cycles. If there was a good place for Blueberries, the People would actually do a burn to preserve the patch. Nearby Birch trees surely profited from this. Interconnectedness is a central concept in the philosophy of the People. No individual species does well without the help of other healthy species. Like Blueberries, Birch do not compete well with invading trees. The burning also helps the nearby Jack Pine who simply cannot reproduce without fire.

The Kirtland Warbler (spring songbird) will only nest in the Jack Pine trees. If the Jack Pine trees go, the Warbler goes. Then the Earth falls a little short of its full potential, and we do not hear the singing of a beautiful bird. The Birches are in great danger from a root micro-organism. I hope we, the People, can help them. I can't imagine a northern forest without Birch trees.

Drying and Storing Plants

There are many questions about storing herbs, and I will try to answer some of those questions now. First in importance is to dry the plants or roots thoroughly. When dry the leaves are brittle, and they will crumble easily. Take the time before harvesting to inspect the plants. If an insect has chewed or built a home on the leaf, choose a different leaf. With spiders, the brown bag method of drying is effective. Leave the bag open on one end, so as the plants dry the spider can wander out of the bag to find a new home elsewhere. Drying plants is like making hay, as the plants need to be turned every day. I use the beloved brown bags so I can shake them or turn the bag over, rather than turn every plant (clever herbalist trick).

When the plants are dry I transfer them to clean canning jars. These jars are made of glass and have an airtight lid. I caution you not to store plants for medicine in plastic bags or plastic containers, as they always leak the chemicals used to make them. Remember to label the glass jars as soon as you fill them. Crumbled leaves are difficult to identify by smell alone. I use cellophane tape to make certain the labels stay on the jars. I also label the lids to make it easy to find the right jar even if I fill a shelf with herb jars. For best storage, keep the jars away from sunlight, as the light fades the color of the herbs. You want your green herbs to stay deep green.

I keep dry roots, seeds and bark for up to two years. Dry leaves and stems I renew every year. If I have gathered a little too much of a leafy plant, then I mix the excess plant into my Kinnik to become part of the Prayers. For the People of the Great Lakes there was only one Law, "Do Not Waste."

I hope this journal is only a beginning of your relationship with plants and trees. The Green Ones are the intermediary for us with the living Earth. Plants absorb the energy of the Sun and transform the rocks and minerals of this planet into living tissue. They do this so that they may live. They share themselves so we also can live. The Plants are willing to share their Medicines, and we need only ask in a good way. We must promise to see to the "ongoing of the Plants." Let these Wild Plants be a part of where you live, they are fine neighbors, and they are beautiful.

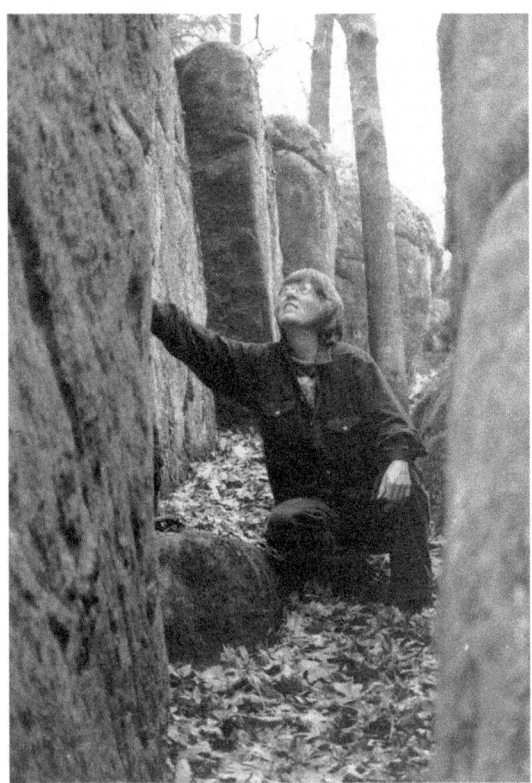

Judith Meister is a field biologist living in Madison, Wisconsin. She studied fifteen years with a traditional herbalist giving her a solid foundation to Native American philosophy and medicinal plant use. She is also the author of a novel, *Their Time of Learning*.

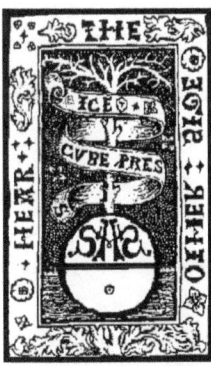 Ice Cube Books began publishing in 1993 to focus on how to live with the natural world and to better understand how people can best live together in the communities they share and inhabit. Since this time, we've been recognized by a number of well-known writers, including Gary Snyder, Gene Logsdon, Wes Jackson, Patricia Hampl, Greg Brown, Jim Harrison, Annie Dillard, Ken Burns, Kathleen Norris, Janisse Ray, Alison Deming, Richard Rhodes, Michael Pollan, and Barry Lopez. We've published a number of well-known authors as well, including Mary Swander, Jim Heynen, Mary Pipher, Bill Holm, Connie Mutel, John T. Price, Carol Bly, Marvin Bell, Debra Marquart, Ted Kooser, Stephanie Mills, Bill McKibben, and Paul Gruchow. As well, we have won several publishing awards over the last seventeen years. Check out our books at our web site, with booksellers, or at museum shops, then discover why we strive to "hear the other side."

Ice Cube Press (est. 1993)
205 N Front Street
North Liberty, Iowa 52317-9302
steve@icecubepress.com
www.icecubepress.com

planting hearts and souls with
hugs & kisses & then away we go to
Fenna Marie-o & Laura Lee-o

Printed in the USA
CPSIA information can be obtained
at www.ICGtesting.com
LVHW091207060624
782367LV00001B/61